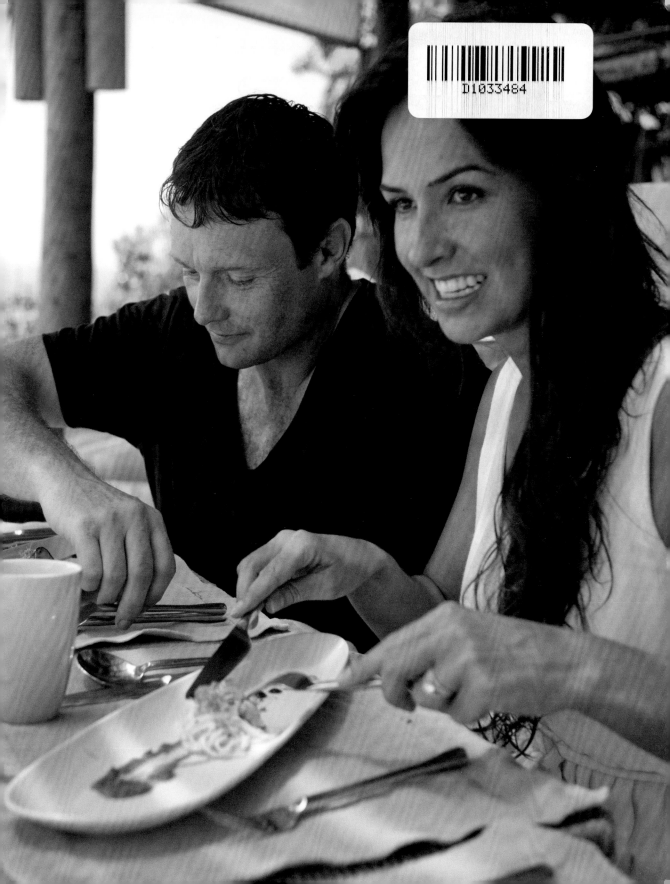

Published in 2014 by Kyle Books
www.kylebooks.com
Distributed by National Book Network
4501 Forbes Blvd., Suite 200
Lanham, MD 20706
Phone: (800) 462-6420
Fax: (800) 338-4550
customercare@nbnbooks.com

First published in Great Britain in 2012 by
Kyle Cathie Limited

ISBN 978-1-909487-05-5

Editor Judith Hannam
Design Dale Walker
Model Christiane Duigan
Clothes by Grace and Favour at b.PR
Recipe home economy and styling Emma Jane Frost
Editor Judith Hannam
Copy editor Anne Newman
Proofreader Anna Irvin
Production Nic Jones, David Hearn, and Lisa Pinnell
Library of Congress Control No. 2013948544

Printed in China

Disclaimer

The information and advice contained in this book are
intended as a general guide. Neither the author nor the
publishers can be held responsible for claims arising from
the inappropriate use of any remedy or exercise regime.
Do not attempt self-diagnosis or self-treatment for serious
or long-term conditions before consulting a medical
professional or qualified practitioner. Do not begin any
exercise program or undertake any self-treatment while
taking other prescribed drugs or receiving therapy
without first seeking professional guidance. Always seek
medical advice if any symptoms persist.

James Duigan

CLEAN
&LEAN DIET
COOKBOOK

OVER 100 DELICIOUS
HEALTHY RECIPES WITH
A 14-DAY MENU PLAN

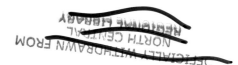

James Duigan, world-renowned wellness guru and

co-owner of Bodyism, London's premier health and

wellness facility, is one of the world's top personal trainers.

His glittering client list includes Elle Macpherson,

Rosie Huntington-Whiteley, and Hugh Grant.

KYLE BOOKS

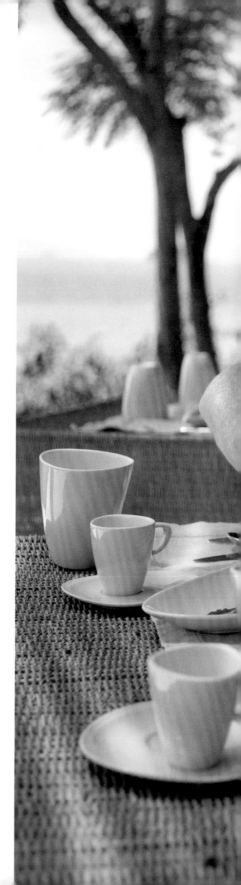

CLEAN
&LEAN DIET
COOKBOOK

OVER 100 DELICIOUS HEALTHY RECIPES WITH A 14-DAY MENU PLAN

JAMES DUIGAN
with Maria Lally

PHOTOGRAPHY BY
SEBASTIAN ROOS AND
CHARLIE RICHARDS

KYLE BOOKS

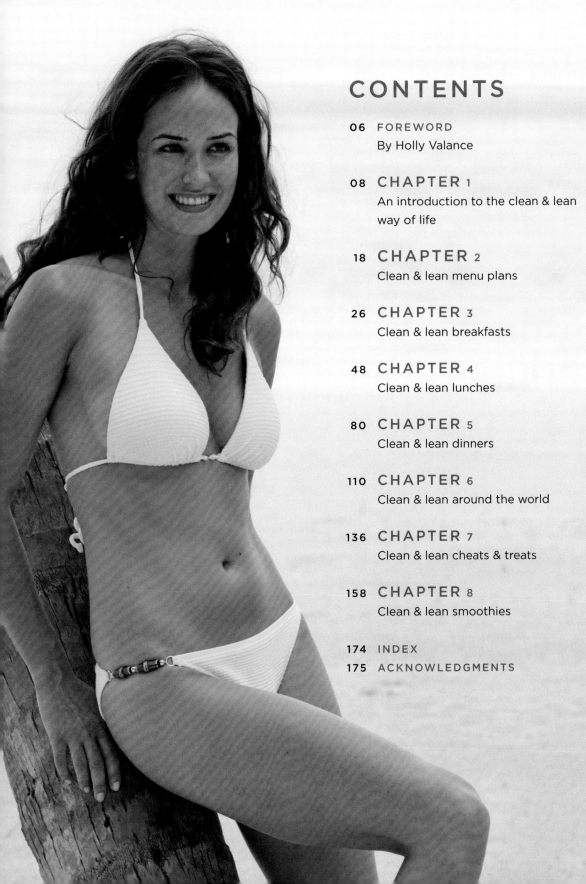

CONTENTS

by Holly Valance

Ask me to do something, and I probably won't. Ask me not to, and I'll hop to it! It's always been that way! So when James and I started out on our first training session I figured I had another guy who'd poo poo everything I've always done, and try to make me do things I've never really been interested in doing to begin with. Guess what? I was wrong. Which I've only been once before, obviously.

~

Becoming Clean & Lean is the simplest, most enjoyable lifestyle choice I've made, and the only one I've actually stuck to. And it's been easy. Clean & Lean eating is common sense, and your body doesn't have to go through any torturous reactions—as it does with silly fads—to get results.

~

My training sessions are really enjoyable. My body has responded how I always wanted it to, but never did before. With Clean & Lean James has really tapped into how we can function at the highest levels realistic to our busy lifestyles. That's why you'll get results. And that's why you'll stick to it. It really is that easy.

~

You need to be healthy first and foremost. Inside and out. And the hardest part is actually your head. Once you decide you want to be at your optimum, whatever that may be for you, focus on that, and not on what the Barbie girl who's been retouched within an inch of her life looks like.

~

So, remember:

We can't all be supermodels. We can all be Clean & Lean. There's an opportunity through exercise and diet to create a longer healthier life, a calmer mind, and better existence for ourselves. And that's what this is really about. Living life better!

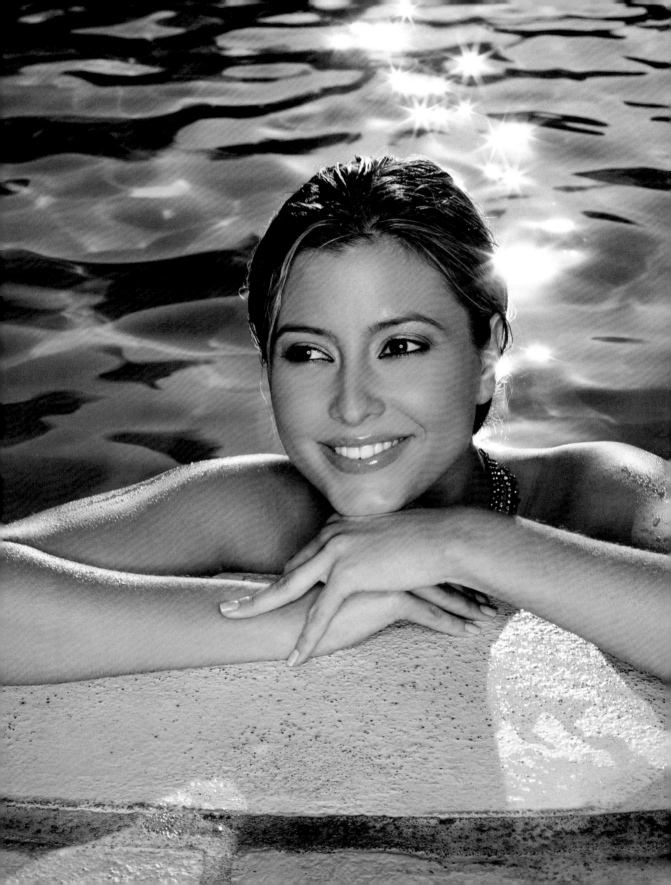

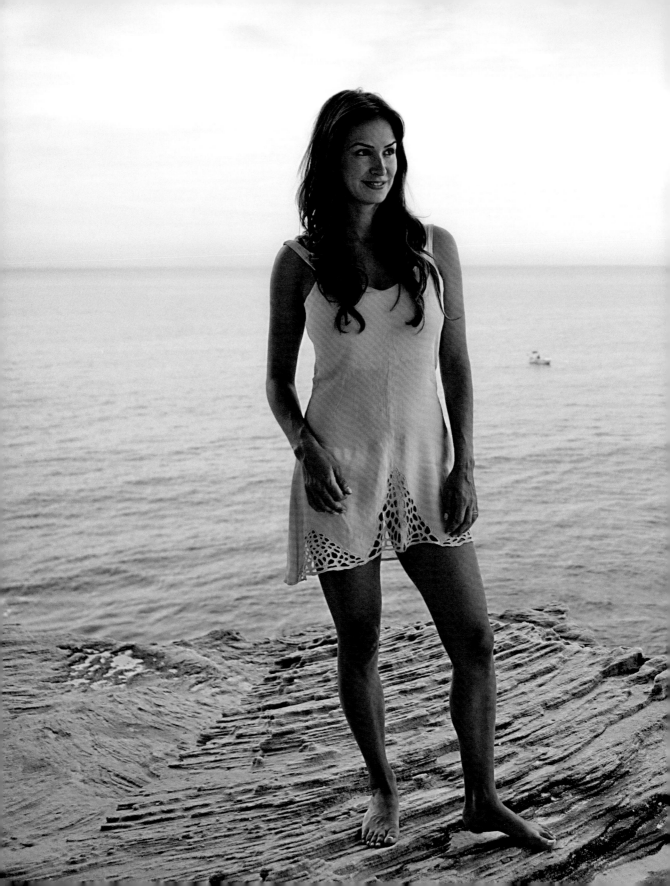

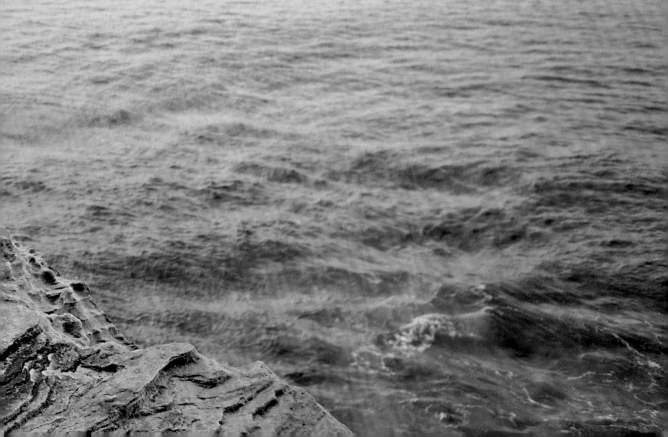

CHAPTER 1

INTRODUCTION

THIS CHAPTER WILL REVEAL:

1. WHY YOU NEED TO BE CLEAN TO BE LEAN

2. THE EXCUSES THAT ARE STOPPING YOU FROM BECOMING SLIM AND HEALTHY

3. HOW OUR COVER GIRL GOT HER BODY

"Thousands of people have changed their lives by becoming Clean & Lean. It's a term I came up with to describe the perfect body: 'Clean' of fattening toxins and 'lean' and healthy as a result. No more excuses. NOW is the time to change your life."

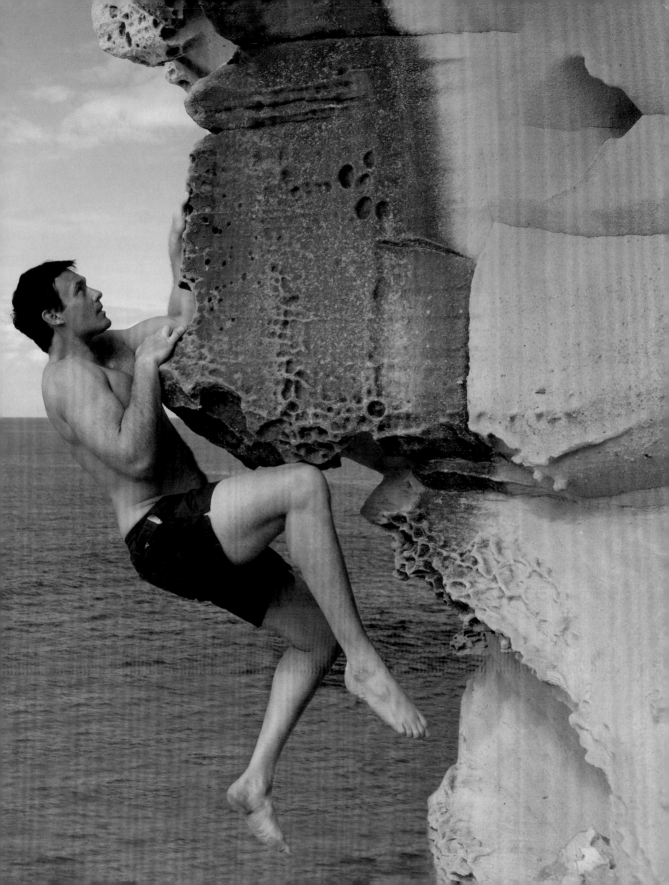

AN INTRODUCTION FROM JAMES

Since writing *Clean & Lean*, my wife Christiane and I have been overwhelmed by the inspirational stories we have read from people whose health, bodies, and lives have been transformed by the books. So the first thing I want to say to the thousands of you all over the world who have shared your beautiful stories and asked me for more Clean & Lean recipes is: thank you. It is because of you that I have written this book.

I love food! Christiane and I start talking about lunch before we finish breakfast, and my happiest moments are when I am eating good food with family and friends. But I also understand that we all have a complicated relationship with food, and often, our behaviors are driven by things that happened in our childhood—trauma, abuse, self-punishment, and scarcity, to name a few. Let me share a little bit of my own story with you now, in the hope that it might help somebody.

I grew up in quite a poor home where, sometimes, there was no food on the table. Other times, there wasn't even a table. There was, however, lots of love, laughter, and singing and, no matter how bad things were, my dad was a superhero and always made things OK. So I feel very lucky to have had the things I had, but being hungry sucked. It is an enduring and powerful memory from my childhood and it affected my relationship with food for years without me ever knowing. I never understood why I ate the way I did—why I would binge eat until I felt sick and could hardly move. And, regardless of what I'd already eaten, I could never leave anything on my plate. I guess all this came from a deep belief that food was scarce and that I didn't know where my next meal was coming from. Now that I understand what was driving this behavior, I can tell the hungry little glutton inside me that there is plenty of food and that I don't need to eat everything I see. Recognizing this has helped me to deal with it, and I hope this may get some of you thinking about any of your own eating habits that aren't working for you and why they happen in the first place.

One of my other enduring memories is of my mother's beautiful cooking. She could make anything taste great and she instilled in me a deep appreciation for good food cooked well. We grew a lot of our own vegetables and she always tried to get organic food whenever she could in whichever town or city we were living in at the time. She

also noticed that whenever I had sugar I would throw a tantrum and run around in circles for twenty minutes, then cry for an hour (that still happens to this day), so my childhood was largely sugar-free, apart from the epic binges I managed at grandparents' and friends' houses. Although at the time being the only sugar-free kid didn't feel so good, I'm grateful for it now, as I feel it has played a big part in me feeling so healthy as an adult. My relationship with food is now one of unconditional love: I love food and food loves me.

So this is not a diet book. Many books about getting in shape are anti-food, but this one is different. I want to help you change your relationship with food and see it as something to be enjoyed while you're relaxed and happy, not something that stirs up feelings of shame, guilt, and despair, leaving you feeling miserable and helpless. I want you to love food, and to find as much joy in it as Christiane and I do.

Food is one of our main life sources. It nourishes us, keeps us strong, and can make us look and feel amazing. It lifts our mood and our energy levels. When you view it in this way, and eat nourishing foods that are good for you, the weight will drop off and you'll feel amazing. But when you view food as the enemy, as something that is "bad" for you, you'll remain stuck in that all-too-common cycle of deprivation and "reward"—the reward being a binge on fatty, sugary foods that gives you a quick, fleeting high followed by a feeling of sickness, tiredness, and, ultimately, guilt and shame. Then the cycle of deprivation will start all over again.

This book features some of my own favorite recipes, and I've asked some of my friends—including Elle Macpherson, Rosie Huntington-Whiteley, and Hugh Grant—plus my brilliant team at Bodyism to share with you some of theirs too.

I also talk about the attitudes of other cultures toward food. I've traveled extensively and have picked up tips on what works from countries all over the world. In Australia, for example, where I come from, eating is a very sociable activity; we love our meat and vegetables, and enjoy BBQs and eating outside. You can follow the Clean & Lean rules wherever you go and still enjoy your food, if you take note of what I say in the following chapters. Plus, there are delicious recipes from all over the world for you to try.

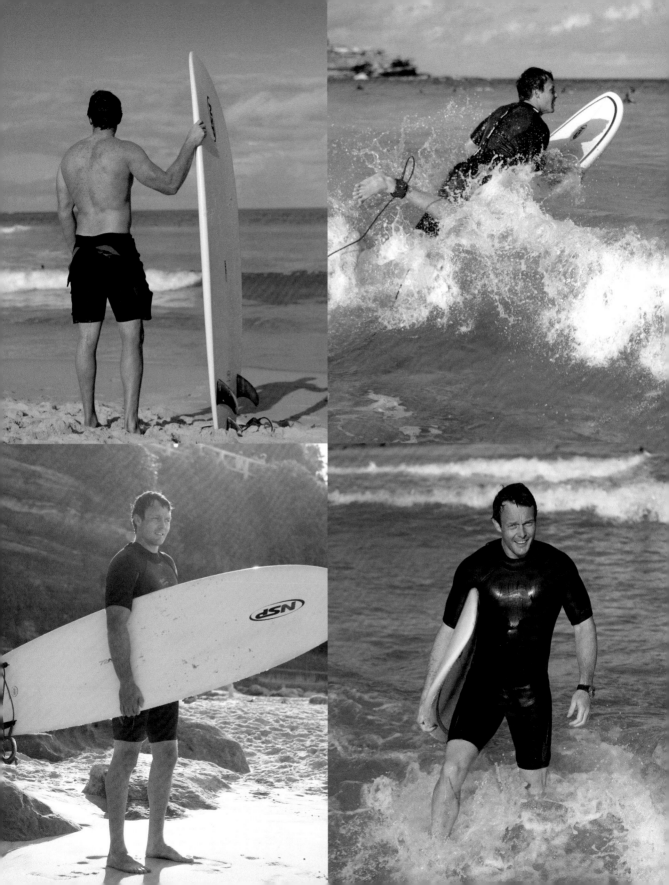

A VERY QUICK REMINDER ABOUT THE CLEAN & LEAN REGIME

A body can never be lean unless it's clean. That's the first principle, and it's toxins, which are stored in the fat cells, that you need to avoid. If you're dieting, but toxic, your body will lose fat, but the toxins will have nowhere to go other than back into your system. This is why you often soon feel terrible after starting a diet—tired, lethargic, and headachey. Your body quickly decides it doesn't like feeling this way and therefore holds on to fat in order to store toxins, and so the cycle continues. If you're toxic, you'll always struggle to lose weight and, ironically, many diets make you more toxic with all their low-fat/high-sugar advice. However, if you stick to "clean" foods that are toxin-free, unprocessed, and close to their natural state, you'll lose weight easily and keep it off.

WHAT ARE CLEAN FOODS?

✳ They haven't changed much from their natural state. For example, that apple in your fruit bowl looks like it did when it was hanging on the tree, yet potato chips don't resemble potatoes. That's because they've been processed.
✳ They don't have any added artificial flavor.
✳ They don't last for months on the shelf. Clean foods develop mold or go bad quite quickly because they're natural and not packed with life-lengthening preservatives.
✳ They don't have long lists of ingredients, many of which you can't even pronounce, let alone recognize.
✳ They don't list sugar among their first three ingredients—sugars usually end in "ose," e.g. fructose, sucrose, glucose.

WHAT ARE THE CLEAN & LEAN RULES?

Here's a quick run-through of the rules.

SUGAR – NOT SO SWEET

Sugar makes you fat. It converts to fat quicker than fat itself because it raises your insulin levels, which causes fat storage. Studies show that 40 percent of the sugar you eat is converted straight to fat, and that's in a slim person. If you're already overweight, up to 60 percent is converted straight to fat and stored around your stomach, waist, and hips. Put simply—if you eat sugar every day, you'll always struggle to lose weight.

Sugar also leaches vitamins from your body, and a body starved of vitamins is a hungry one. That's one of the main reasons that overweight people are always hungry—they don't eat enough vitamin-rich food and are malnourished. It also makes you tired and weakens your immune system. Lots of so-called "diet" or "low-fat" foods and drinks are packed with sugar because, yes, it is technically low in fat, but the sugar converts to fat.

ANOTHER KEY CLEAN & LEAN RULE IS TO CUT OUT CRAP

Cut the CRAP* (that's *Caffeine, Refined sugar, Alcohol, and Processed foods) ©
Caffeine is OK in small doses. One or two cups of coffee a day won't do much harm. Some studies suggest it can even help with fat burning, especially if you drink the organic kind. Green tea also contains caffeine and you can have up to six cups of this a day (any more will affect your sleep). The trouble with too much coffee (which contains more caffeine than green tea) is that it puts stress on your system. When we're stressed, we release a hormone called cortisol which encourages our body to cling to fat. So to sum up, one or two coffees = fine; too many = a fat middle.

I've already talked about refined sugar—in cakes, cookies, "diet" foods and drinks, chocolate, and fizzy drinks—so let's move on to alcohol now. Alcohol is full of sugar and, as a result, it makes you fat around the middle. It also stimulates the production of the hormone estrogen, which promotes fat storage around your waist and tummy. Remember, too, that the liver is a fat-burning organ so when it's processing alcohol, it stops burning fat. In short, alcohol leaves you squishy around the middle.

Processed foods go against every Clean & Lean rule there is. The less a food has been altered, the "cleaner" it is, which is good news for our waistlines. Clean foods are very close to—if not the same as—their natural state. Processed foods, on the other hand, are usually made in factories, stripped of their natural goodness, and pumped full of man-made preservatives and additives to make them look appetizing and last longer. So stay away from bread, pasta, and white rice, some canned foods, pre-made meals, most breakfast cereals, and frozen french fries.

FAT DOESN'T MAKE YOU FAT

Don't be fat phobic! When I talk about fat, I mean good fat—the heart-friendly kind found in nuts, avocados, oily fish, and oils, not bad fat, on the edge of a strip of bacon or other processed meat, or in a pie crust. Good, clean fats should be eaten every day. They encourage your body to burn fat around your middle, and to absorb vitamins and minerals more efficiently. Good fats also reduce sugar cravings, lift your energy levels and ability to concentrate, and keep you full for a long time.

WHERE ARE TOXINS FOUND?

Toxins are found in the following:
* Sugar
* Alcohol
* Fizzy drinks
* Processed foods
* Processed "diet" foods
* Excess caffeine
* Artificial sweeteners
* Food additives
* Preservatives
* Artificial color
* Artificial enhancers, like MSG and many E numbers e.g. E621 is a sneaky way of saying MSG
* Pesticides—wash your fruit and veggies thoroughly

WHAT'S YOUR FOOD HANGOVER?

Food can make you feel really, really good. I'm talking energized, alert, slim, fit, and young. It can make your skin glow and your hair shine. But food can also make you feel really, really bad too. If you eat the wrong types of food, it can make you feel fat, bloated, tired, and guilty. So think about how you want to feel before you next eat.

You see, I don't actually believe that overweight or unhealthy people enjoy their food. Sure, I think they like the look of that chocolate bar, or the smell of fish and chips, but how do they feel after eating it? Pretty bad. I know, because that's what my clients tell me when they speak about their past battles with food. You need to decide whether you want food to make you feel good or bad? It's a simple choice, and I think we both already know the answer, otherwise you wouldn't have picked up this book.

If you do struggle with food, bingeing, or yo-yo dieting, try turning your negative thoughts into positive ones. A very effective strategy for changing your negative habits to positive ones that transform your body and life is to say affirmations and practice visualization. So for example:
Don't think: "I'm fat, I look disgusting, and feel bloated."
Think instead: "I am so slim, healthy, and feel beautiful. Weight loss is effortless and easy."
Don't think: "I can't have that chocolate bar," or, if you just ate a chocolate bar, "I feel guilty for eating that."
Think instead: "I listen to my body and nourish it with only the foods that make me feel amazing and energized. I am safe and all is good."
Don't think: "I haven't got time to make a healthy meal or exercise."
Think instead: "I love and care for my body. Abundance of time and health flows to me."
Or try visualization: at any time of day or when you are drifting off to sleep or waking up, picture your legs, tummy, bottom, arms—your whole body—looking the way you want it to look, and emphasize the sense of how that makes you feel. Do this as regularly as you remember.

So change your thoughts and beliefs and you can instantly change your emotional state.

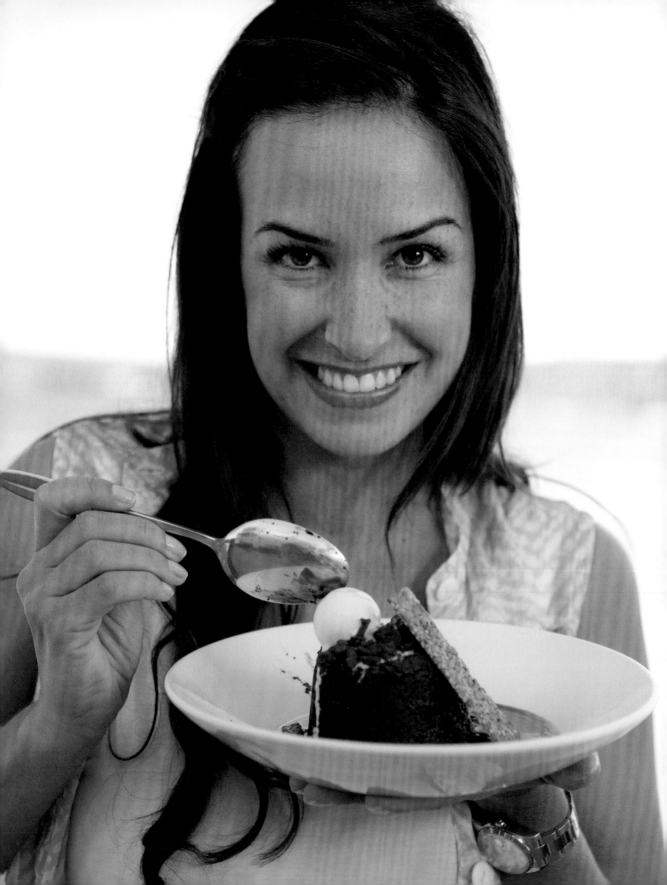

"Eating is my favorite thing to do!"

Our cover girl—and Mrs. James Duigan—Christiane, reveals why changing her relationship with food changed her body:

Since I met James in 2006 I've discovered just how much I love food. James and I love to eat—it's one of our favorite things to do! Whenever we travel abroad we rate the country on the food we eat there and love discovering new dishes and restaurants. In fact, we're such foodies our friends are always asking us for recommendations on where to eat.

Before I met James, I had a very different relationship with food. I ate less than I do now and exercised more. Now I know that I was eating all the wrong types of food for my body like fruit or low-fat yogurts. I had only salad on a plate and drank skim milk and diet drinks. I was hungry a lot of the time—but heavier. I often felt guilty when I did eat fatty foods, so I would wolf them down, but then feel even worse afterward. And so the cycle would continue...

Then I met James and he told me about Clean & Lean. No food was off limits, but I had to listen to my body and let it be my own personal nutritionist. So if a food made me feel tired, heavy, gassy, or bloated, I avoided it. If I wanted some lasagna or pasta, I'd have it, but I'd eat it slowly and savor every mouthful. I wouldn't feel guilty—I would enjoy it but, crucially, I would stop when I was full or starting to feel uncomfortable. By just enjoying the food and feeling good about what I was eating, the weight fell off and I haven't gained a pound since.

The key to being slim is to enjoy your food. Any transformation that happens in the body, happens in your mind first. What you are thinking and feeling will be reflected in your body. You have to try it to believe it!

James, we all can't thank you enough. Hundreds of people have written in after reading your books to express their gratitude to you for the transformation and impact you have made on their lives. You have inspired so many people to make positive changes to their health, bodies, and lifestyle. You have always wanted to make a difference in the world and help others and you have done that through your persistent kindness, love, and generosity. From your family, friends, clients, and everyone that has read your books— THANK YOU!

On a personal note, Amor, not only have you changed my life in terms of health, you have brought me so much love and happiness. I have found a love with you like no other and I am so grateful for you, our friendship, and to have you as my husband. My happiest moments are with you, creating our amazing life together since the moment we fell in love over chocolate soup! You're a true inspiration and I'm so proud of you. Thank you, *Te amo muito!!*

christiane

A FINAL WORD

When I was publicizing my first two books, I met lots of readers. One woman was overweight and miserable as a result, but tried to tell me she was "too busy" to do anything about it. She said she didn't have time to prepare her meals. "Fine," I told her. "Just have some pre-cooked chicken or salmon and salad or something easy like an omelet with greens when you get home from work." But she said she didn't have time. When I suggested she try to walk for thirty minutes a day, or try a yoga class every now and then, she told me she didn't have time for that either. She was negative and wanted to prove to me she didn't have time to look and feel good. She had kids and a busy job, she kept saying. Then another woman—who was slim and healthy looking—said to the two of us: "I've got three kids too, and a job, and a house to run. But I make time to eat the right stuff and move around a bit when I get the chance." This encounter made me realize that some people look for obstacles when it comes to getting in shape. Instead of thinking you can't do it, know that you can. You just have to decide whether you want to look and feel slim and healthy or you don't. It's a choice, and only you can make it.

This book is a celebration of food. So read and enjoy all the tasty recipes I've put together here for you. I want you to have fun, to feel good, and to share that with the people you love. Let me know what you think!

James

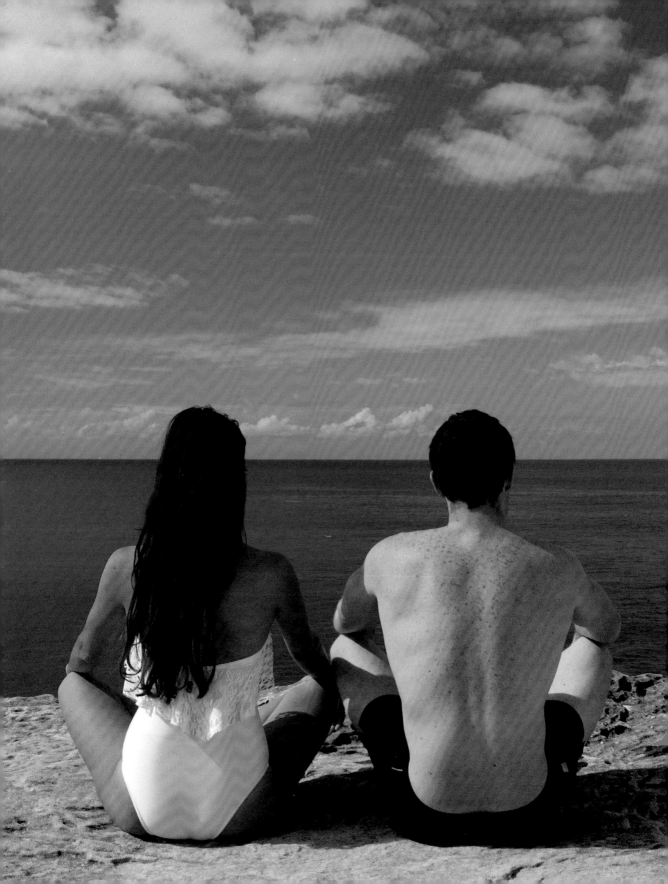

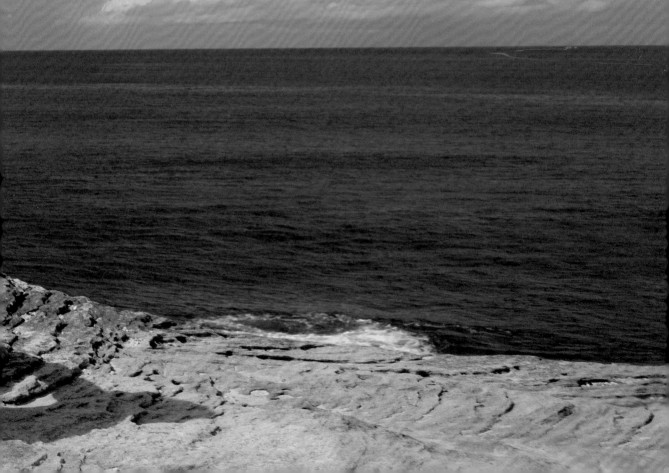

CHAPTER 2

CLEAN AND LEAN MENU PLANS

THIS CHAPTER WILL REVEAL:

1. YOUR PICK 'N' MIX MEAL PLANNER

2. THE 14-DAY MENU PLAN

YOUR PICK 'N' MIX MEAL PLANNER

To prove just how easy the Clean & Lean diet is, I've devised a Pick 'n' Mix chart. It contains three lists of different foods (protein, vegetables, and "flavor") plus a list of cooking methods. All you need to do is pick your favorite protein, your favorite vegetables, favorite flavor, and cook it using your preferred cooking method.

Guide...

1 With your protein, just pick one and have an amount roughly the size of the palm of your hand or a deck of playing cards.

2 With the vegetables, feel free to pick as many different types—and as much—as you like.

3 Feel free to add a small handful of nuts and/or beans or lentils to your meal. It will fill you up and help keep those snack cravings from sneaking up on you later.

A NOTE FOR VEGETARIANS

If you're a vegetarian, feel free to substitute the proteins I've suggested for your usual non-meat source (for example, eggs, beans, lentils, tofu, etc). As for cheese, go for hard white cheeses such as feta and goat cheese. Avoid the heavily processed cheeses that are bright yellow or come in slices and go for the best quality, organic cheese you can afford.

PROTEIN	VEGETABLES	FLAVOR	HOW TO COOK
✳ Any fish	✳ Broccoli	✳ Olive oil	✳ Broil
✳ Chicken	✳ Kale	✳ Flax oil	✳ Bake
✳ Turkey	✳ Spinach	✳ Garlic	✳ Steam
✳ Shrimp	✳ Green beans	✳ Herbs, fresh and dry	✳ Sauté
✳ Veal	✳ Asparagus	✳ Mustard seeds	✳ Stir-fry
✳ Lamb	✳ Arugula	✳ Lemons	✳ Barbecue
✳ Beef	✳ Cucumber	✳ Limes	✳ Blanch
✳ Duck	✳ Zucchini	✳ Chile	
✳ Eggs	✳ Leeks	✳ Ginger	**TRY TO AVOID**
✳ Avocado	✳ Peas	✳ Chamomile	✳ Frying
	✳ Bok choy	✳ Passionflower	✳ Boiling
	✳ Beets		✳ Microwaving
	✳ Bell peppers		
	✳ Sweet potato		
	✳ Eggplant		
	✳ Carrots		
	✳ Mushrooms		

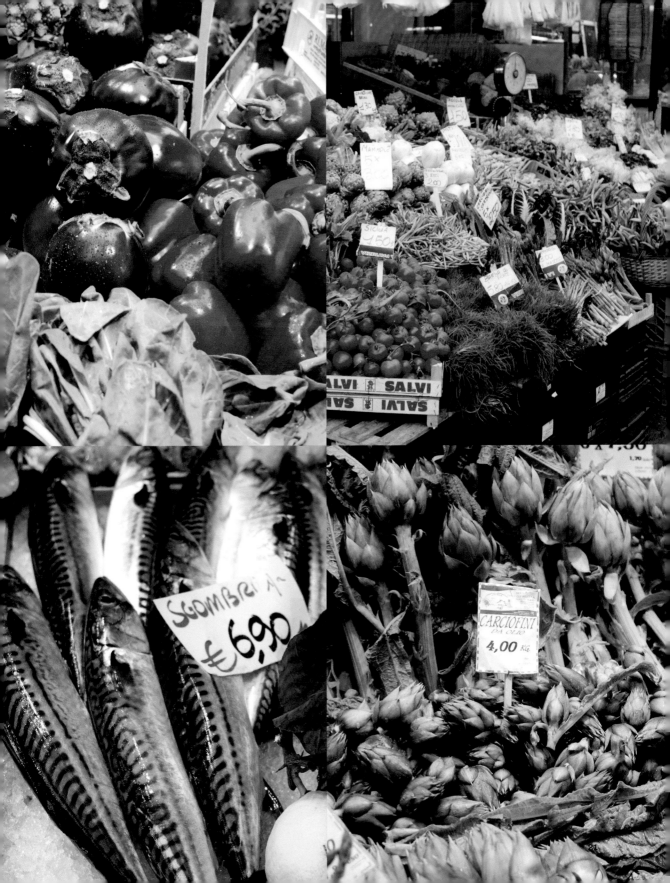

THE 14-DAY EATING PLAN

When you feel ready to start, follow this 14-day plan. It's best to start on a weekend, when you have more time on your hands to get everything ready. Plus you won't feel so stressed or rushed, which will mean you'll be less likely to supplement the plan with a quick coffee or a mid-afternoon chocolate bar.

You can swap meals around (have Day 1 breakfast on Day 2, for example), but try to stick to the plan as much as possible. You shouldn't feel hungry, but if you do, just increase your green vegetable portions and make sure you're drinking enough water (at least 8 glasses of still, filtered water a day).

Where possible (and if you can afford it), go for organic ingredients—especially when it comes to eggs (free-range are also good) and meat

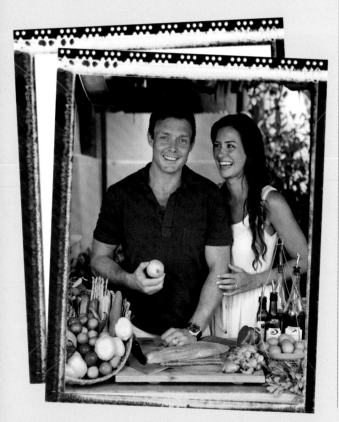

DAY 1

Breakfast: Omelet, with your choice of ingredients from the list on p. 42

Snack, mid-morning: 3½oz chicken breast and ¼ avocado

Lunch: Elle's kale and goat cheese salad (p. 60)

Snack, mid-afternoon: 2 hard-boiled eggs and ½ cucumber, sliced

Dinner: Seared sirloin with arugula and watercress salad (p. 96)

DAY 2

Breakfast: Perfect oatmeal with berries, yogurt, and almonds (p. 38)

Snack, mid-morning: 3½oz turkey and 5 walnuts

Lunch: Quiche with brown rice crust (p. 67)—a great lunch option as it can be made the night before and eaten cold

Snack, mid-afternoon: 3½oz sliced salmon with ¼ avocado

Dinner: Seared wasabi and sesame tuna with chile green beans (p. 96)

WHAT IS 3½OZ?

If you don't have scales to weigh your portions, here's a rough guide to the measurements given in the 14-day plan:

3½oz chicken = two thirds the size of a regular breast or the palm of your hand (minus fingers)

3½oz smoked salmon = the size of your outstretched hand

3½oz beef tenderloin = the size of a tennis ball

DAY 3	DAY 4	DAY 5	DAY 6
Breakfast: Green smoothie (p. 169)	**Breakfast:** Poached eggs with asparagus and smoked salmon (p. 41)	**Breakfast:** Elle's quick scrambled eggs (p. 59)	**Breakfast:** Coconut granola (p. 35)
Snack, mid-morning: 3½oz salmon and 6 pecans	**Snack, mid-morning:** 3½oz chicken breast and 12 cashews	**Snack, mid morning:** 3½oz turkey slices with 5 hazelnuts	**Snack, mid-morning:** 3½oz sliced chicken breast with ½ red bell pepper
Lunch: Crunchy Cambodian-style beef salad (p. 70)—again, another great recipe to eat cold for lunch	**Lunch:** Clean & Lean wrap (p. 73)	**Lunch:** Green super salad (p. 69)	**Lunch:** Red and yellow salad with mackerel (p. 68)
Snack, mid-afternoon: 3½oz cooked shrimp with ½ yellow bell pepper	**Snack, mid-afternoon:** 3½oz turkey slices with ½ green bell pepper, sliced	**Snack, mid-afternoon:** 3½oz beef slices and ¼ cucumber, sliced	**Snack, mid-afternoon:** 3½oz chicken breast and ½ sliced tomato
Dinner: Grilled cajun chicken (p. 99)	**Dinner:** Lamb cutlets with chermoula dip and roast zucchini (p. 105)	**Dinner:** Whole baked sea bass (p. 92)	**Dinner:** Broiled chicken or turkey with radicchio salad (p. 88)

*top tip

Poaching doesn't require any oil or fat and the result is a succulent, tender chicken

DAY 7	DAY 8	DAY 9	DAY 10
Breakfast: Buckwheat pancakes (p. 32)	**Breakfast:** Scrambled eggs, smoked salmon, and asparagus (p. 45)	**Breakfast:** Goat cheese and egg white omelet (p. 42)	**Breakfast:** Morning booster smoothie (p. 167)
Snack, mid-morning: 3½oz chicken breast and 6 pecans	**Snack, mid-morning:** 3½oz salmon with ½ red bell pepper, sliced	**Snack, mid-morning:** 3½oz turkey breast and ¼ avocado	**Snack, mid-morning:** 3½oz chicken breast and 12 cashews
Lunch: Hugh's cold lamb salad (p. 68)	**Lunch:** Clean & lean lettuce wrap (p. 73)	**Lunch:** Green super salad with broiled chicken (p. 69)	**Lunch:** Clean & lean lettuce wrap with chicken, tomato, and avocado (p. 73)
Snack, mid-afternoon: 3½oz chicken breast and ½ sliced tomato	**Snack, mid-afternoon:** 3½oz turkey with a portion of steamed green beans	**Snack, mid-afternoon:** 3½oz turkey with ¼ cucumber, sliced	**Snack, mid-afternoon:** 3½oz chicken breast with ½ yellow bell pepper
Dinner: Rosie's roast chicken (p. 106)	**Dinner:** Turkey burgers (p. 106)	**Dinner:** Balinese steamed fish (p. 118)	**Dinner:** Lamb steak with smashed peas (p. 102)

*it's easy

Good healthy habits are a choice and once they are part of your lifestyle, they will last you a lifetime

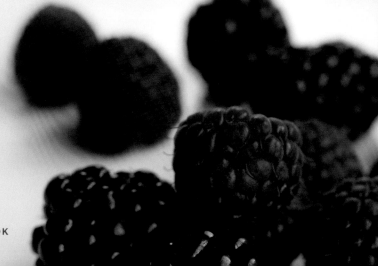

DAY 11

Breakfast: Poached eggs with spinach and mushrooms (p. 41)

Snack, mid-morning: 3½oz turkey and 4 macadamia nuts

Lunch: Hugh's cold lamb salad (p. 68)

Snack, mid-afternoon: 3½oz salmon with ½ green pepper, sliced

Dinner: Chicken skewers (p. 74)

DAY 12

Breakfast: Turkey with avocado, goat cheese, and tomato

Snack, mid-morning: 3½oz beef slices and 5 walnuts

Lunch: Beluga Salad (p. 64)

Snack, mid-afternoon: 3½oz sliced turkey breast with ¼ avocado

Dinner: Grilled chicken or turkey with radicchio salad (p. 88)

DAY 13

Breakfast: Scrambled eggs with shrimp and spinach (p. 59)

Snack, mid morning: 3½oz chicken slices with 5 hazelnuts

Lunch: Gazpacho (p. 55)

Snack, mid-afternoon: 2 hard-boiled eggs and ½ cucumber, sliced

Dinner: Grilled cajun chicken (p. 99)

DAY 14

Breakfast: Coconut granola (p. 35)

Snack, mid-morning: 3½oz turkey with 5 Brazil nuts

Lunch: Clean & lean lettuce wrap (p. 73)

Snack, mid-afternoon: 3½oz turkey breast and ¼ cucumber, sliced

Dinner: French Nicoise salad (p. 131)

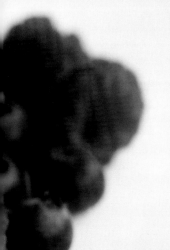

*top tip
Stick this plan on your fridge as a constant reminder—then you won't be tempted to stray

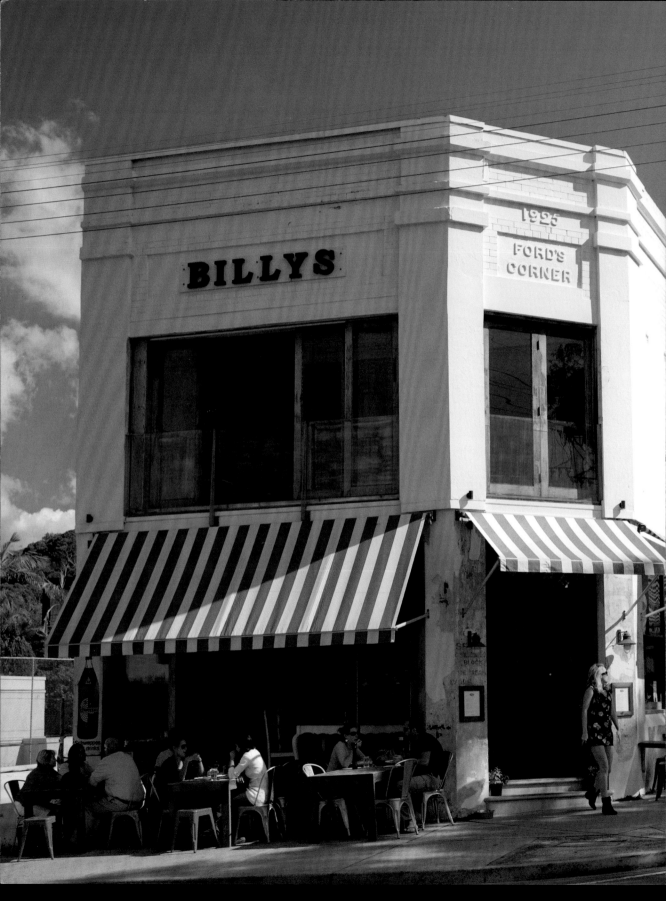

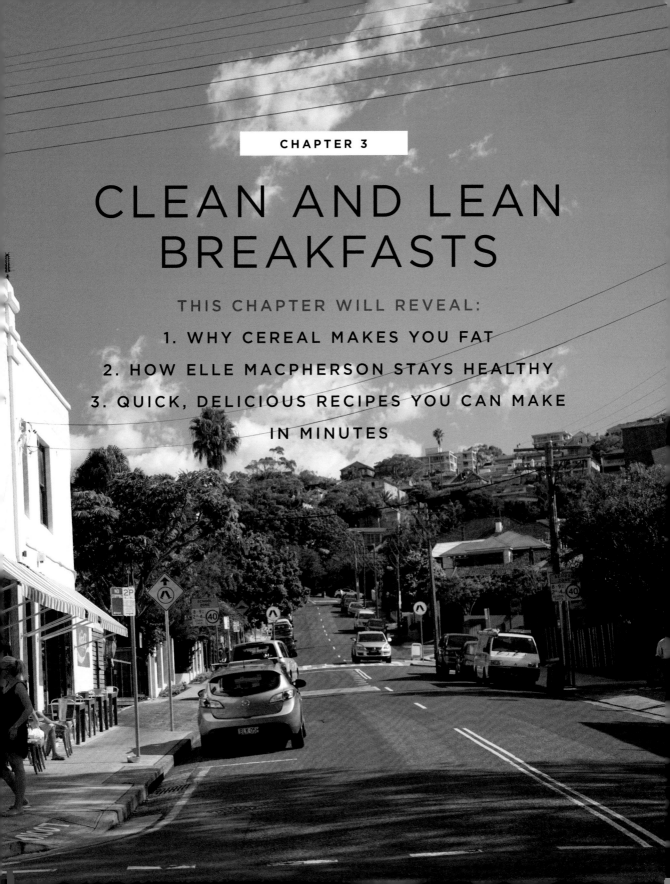

CHAPTER 3

CLEAN AND LEAN BREAKFASTS

THIS CHAPTER WILL REVEAL:

1. WHY CEREAL MAKES YOU FAT

2. HOW ELLE MACPHERSON STAYS HEALTHY

3. QUICK, DELICIOUS RECIPES YOU CAN MAKE IN MINUTES

One of the most important parts of the Clean & Lean regime is to have a good breakfast. What you eat for breakfast determines how your body deals with fat for the whole day, so it's very important to get this meal right. The right breakfast will lift your mood and energy levels and will turn your body into a fat-burning machine for the rest of the day. But if you get it wrong, you'll crave sugar all day and your energy levels and mood will sink fast.

My perfect breakfast is some clean and lean protein in the form of organic fish, eggs, chicken, or even some steak. I cook it the night before and have it cold in the morning with some green beans or broccoli. This leaves me feeling bulletproof. Chicken and green beans for breakfast? Yes, it sounds crazy, but once you get your head around it, you'll realize it's the best thing you can have.

Marketing people have programmed us into picking one of two options for breakfast—two slices of toast with a processed topping or a bowl of sugary cereal with little goodness. Possibly an omelet or scrambled eggs (which are great by the way) as a treat.

But cereal is just about the worst breakfast imaginable. It's over-processed, often full of sugar, and contains zero protein, except possibly the milk. The sugary ones aimed at kids are the worst, but the so-called healthy ones aren't much better. Oatmeal is the only one that's good—have it with nuts, seeds, and berries and you've got a great little breakfast. But as for the rest? Avoid them.

If you—or your children—have cereal in the morning I guarantee you'll be hungry and tired by midday, looking for something sugary to snack on to lift your flagging energy levels. Protein keeps you full, so cereal for breakfast is like putting water in your car instead of petrol. It will fool you for a little while into thinking you've eaten, but you'll be hungry very quickly afterward and will have to snack throughout the day.

Protein and greens, on the other hand, are the perfect combination for breakfast. The protein—be it chicken, fish, eggs—will keep you full for hours and will fire up your metabolism; the greens will provide a hit of vitamins and fiber, which will improve your overall health and well-being. It may take a while to get used to having this sort of thing for breakfast, but just try it for a week and see how amazing you feel. If you don't feel like chicken first thing in the morning, eggs and smoked salmon have always been a popular choice for breakfast, or have a couple of

scrambled eggs with half a sliced avocado. After a while, try out other "protein and green" combinations, like chicken and avocado, smoked salmon with green beans, or—my favorite—steak with broccoli.

THE CLEAN & LEAN BREAKFAST RULES

Here are my breakfast rules:

1 Include protein and greens in your breakfast if you can. But at the very least, you must have some protein in the morning—be it eggs, smoked salmon, meat, cheese, milk, or yogurt.

2 Eat within an hour of waking up to really get your metabolism fired up. If you leave it any longer your body slips into starvation mode and so clings to fat. Eating within an hour of getting up breaks your fast (hence the name), and your body cranks up its fat-burning abilities ready for the day ahead.

3 Take Bodyism BodyBrilliance every morning—a fat-burning blend of antioxidants. Mix two teaspoons with water and have it with your breakfast. Available at www.bodyism.com.

Drink up – how to hydrate at breakfast

In a perfect world, I'd suggest you have some slightly cooled boiled water with a squeeze of fresh lemon juice when you first wake up. It's the perfect drink to hydrate you and detox your system. If you can get into this very quick and simple habit, you'll notice a difference in your energy levels, skin, and hair, and you'll look less bloated. Another good option is a cup of green tea. But at the very least you should be drinking a glass of water as soon as you wake up. Have one by your bed and sip it as you get up.

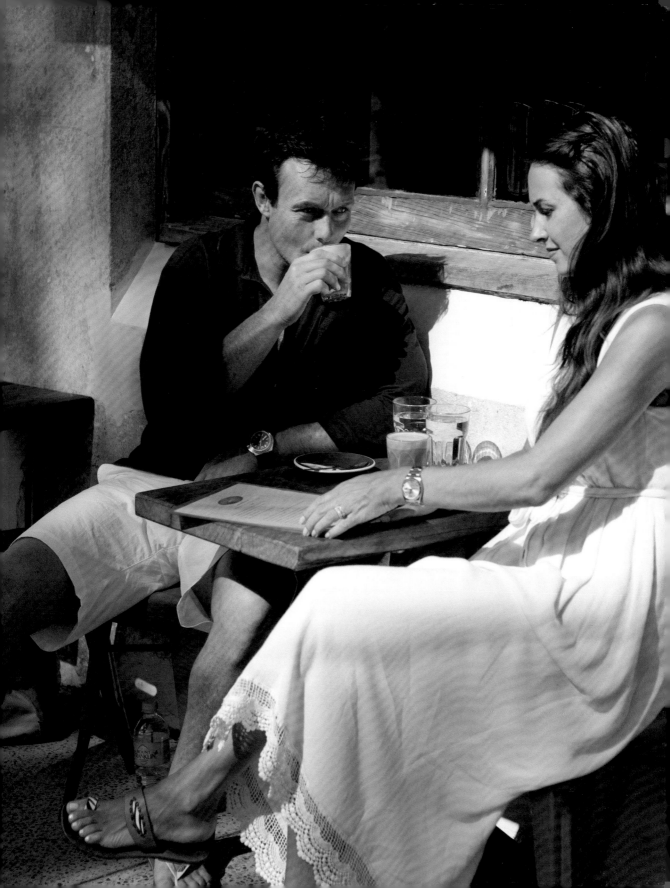

Coffee or tea in the morning is fine. Everyone loves it and I certainly wouldn't advise you not to have it, but have one of the options above first. Just stick to one cup of coffee or tea at breakfast (leaving you free to have another mid-morning or lunchtime). Buy a good-quality, organic coffee or tea and have it with organic full-fat milk, which is better for you than low-fat varieties. If you're eating Clean & Lean overall, you don't need to worry about the extra calories in full-fat milk. I always take it—or even organic cream—in my coffee and I'm slim. Full-fat milk contains more calcium and will keep you fuller for longer. Plus, good natural fats won't make you fat, if the rest of your diet is clean.

Green tea is also great to have every morning. It also contains caffeine, but less so than coffee and many more antioxidants. You can drink up to six cups a day and I tell all my clients to drink it.

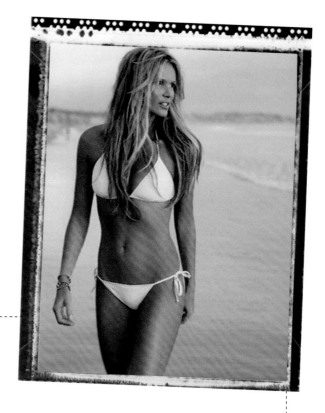

HOW I STAY HEALTHY – BY ELLE MACPHERSON

I've known James for nearly twenty years and I still use his Clean & Lean philosophy to this day. When we started working together he immediately understood that I wanted to maintain a long, lean, healthy body while retaining my femininity and curves. But he also understood that I'm a busy woman—especially after having my two sons—trying to fit in healthy eating with a demanding job and two children. I just don't have the mental energy to be obsessive at the gym or about food.

What works for me is his balanced approach, which results in a healthy, vibrant, and strong body. I choose to forgo quick fixes, drastic regimes, and hours pounding my body in the gym. All I need is the right information and the motivation to do what's required.

As I've gotten older, my body and metabolism, have changed—what worked for me in my 20s and 30s doesn't work for me now. But as always, James and I have worked together to find a solution; nutritional tweaks, along with amazing stress-relieving and body-energizing supplements. James' approach is non-gimmicky and straightforward. He works from the inside out and I'm in the best shape ever because of this. We're both Australian and we love an outdoor lifestyle and the same kinds of food. A true testament to James is that we're still working together after all these years. Why? Because he keeps things relevant and fun—it works! There is literally nobody better in the world than James for getting a woman's body into amazing shape. After all, check out his wife in this book! She's a true testament to the Clean & Lean way of life.

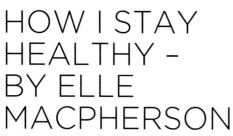

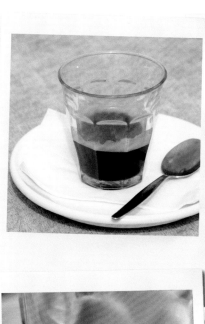
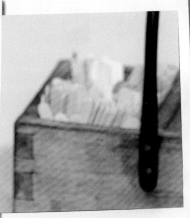
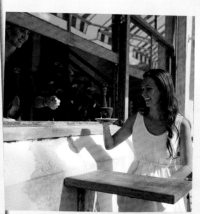
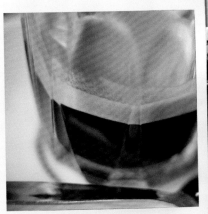
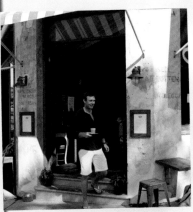
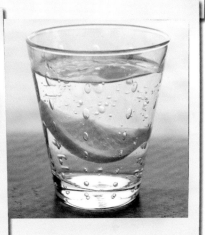
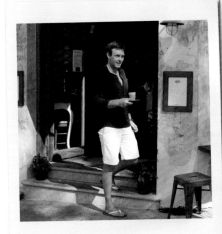
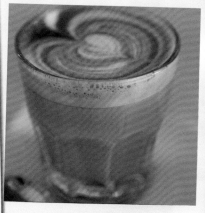
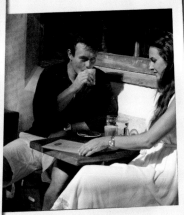

Clean & Lean Oat Pancakes

Serves 2–4

Ingredients
1 cup rolled oats
¾ cup fat-free cottage cheese
4 large eggs
1 teaspoon cinnamon

Method
1. Blend the ingredients in a food processor.
2. Pour a ladleful into a heated pan and cook for 2–3 minutes on each side.

My top breakfasts

My absolute perfect breakfast is sitting in the sun at a café called **Trio** at Bondi Beach, eating boss eggs (the best eggs in the world—they have feta cheese and truffle oil in them) with my beautiful family and my beautiful, gorgeous wife. We sit there and we laugh and listen to the great music the owner plays. **Kensington Square Kitchen** in London does incredible eggs and coffee, and **Gjelina's** in Los Angeles does an incredible whole grain, organic egg sandwich with the yummiest coffee on the West Coast. Then there is **Norma's** in New York that does epic breakfasts that last until lunch time.

*top tip

Berries are rich in antioxidants to detox your system, packed with vitamin C which helps your body deal with stress, and full of fiber which helps to regulate blood-sugar levels

Buckwheat and Blueberry Pancakes

Serves 4

Ingredients
1 cup milk
1 large organic egg
½ cup whole wheat flour
½ cup buckwheat flour
1 cup blueberries
vegetable oil, for cooking
maple syrup, for drizzling

Method
1. In a large bowl, whisk the milk and egg together, then gradually add the flours and whisk well until you have a smooth batter. Stir in the blueberries.

2. In a heavy-bottomed frying pan, heat 1 teaspoon oil. Once hot, spoon in a small ladleful of the batter and keep in a small round shape.

3. After 2–3 minutes, flip and cook for the same amount of time. Repeat until you have roughly 8 pancakes. Serve drizzled with maple syrup.

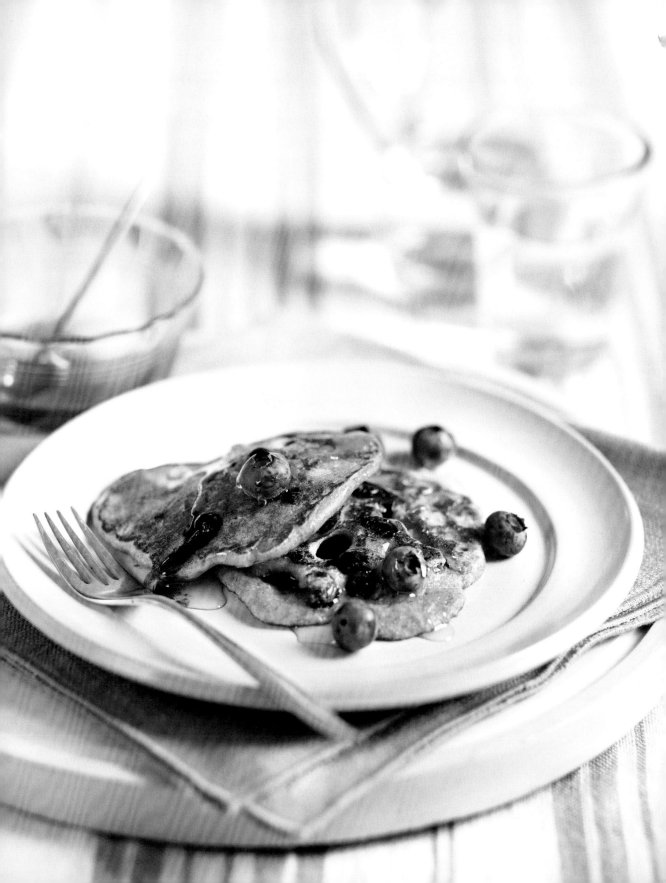

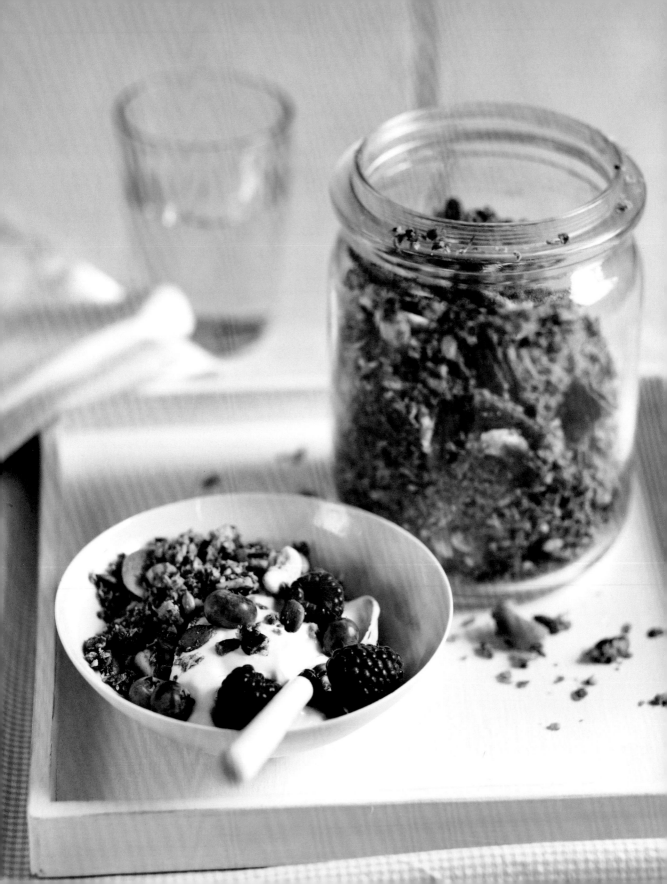

Toasted Pecan and Oat Blueberry Crunch

Serves 4

Ingredients

1¾ cups pecans, chopped
1 cup walnuts, halved
1 cup shredded coconut
2 cups rolled oats
1 teaspoon ground cinnamon
1 cup blueberries
plain organic yogurt, to serve

Method

1. Preheat the oven to 350°F.

2. In large bowl, mix together the nuts, coconut, rolled oats, and cinnamon. Spread onto a baking sheet and toast in the preheated oven for roughly 10 minutes, or until golden, turning halfway through cooking.

3. Let cool, then toss with the blueberries and serve with the yogurt.

*top tip

Swap the walnuts for almonds or pistachios if you want, or combine a delicious mixture of all three

*top tip

You can use any grain you like in this; I often choose a mixture of quinoa flakes and oats

Coconut Granola

Ingredients

6 cups rolled oats
4 tablespoons coconut oil
2 tablespoons ground cinnamon
3 teaspoons vanilla seeds
¼ cup sunflower and pumpkin seeds
2 tablespoons flaxseeds
¼ cup pecans, broken in to small pieces
¼ cup cashews or any nut of your choice
1½ tablespoons toasted or dried coconut

Method

1. Preheat the oven to 375°F and line two baking sheets with parchment paper.

2. Put the oats, 2 tablespoons coconut oil, cinnamon, and vanilla seeds in a bowl and mix well. Spread the mixture evenly onto the prepared baking sheets, then place in the preheated oven. Bake for 20 minutes, checking throughout and turning after 10 minutes.

3. Heat 2 tablespoons coconut oil in a pan and add the seeds, nuts, and coconut. Lightly toast until slightly golden, then set aside to cool.

4. When everything is cooled, mix together and place in a glass jar or storage container. Then this is ready for you to have as a healthy breakfast with some plain organic yogurt, to use as a topping for crumbles, or to add some crunch to some berries. Enjoy!

Gluten-free Sprouted Bread with Smoked Salmon and Avocado

Serves 4

Ingredients
4 slices gluten-free sprouted grain bread
7oz smoked salmon
2 avocados, halved and sliced
black pepper
1 lemon, quartered

Method
1. Preheat the broiler.

2. Warm the bread slices under the preheated broiler and serve with the smoked salmon, avocado slices, black pepper, and lemon wedges.

*top tip
If you don't have any time to make breakfast, just grab half an avocado, slice it up, and have it on a few whole grain crackers or oatcakes

Mackerel with Rye Bread

Serves 1

Ingredients
1 mackerel fillet
¼ cup cottage cheese
juice of ½ lemon
sea salt and freshly ground black pepper, to taste
a slice of rye bread

Method
Mix the mackerel, cottage cheese, lemon, and salt and pepper together and serve on rye bread. This is also great as a snack.

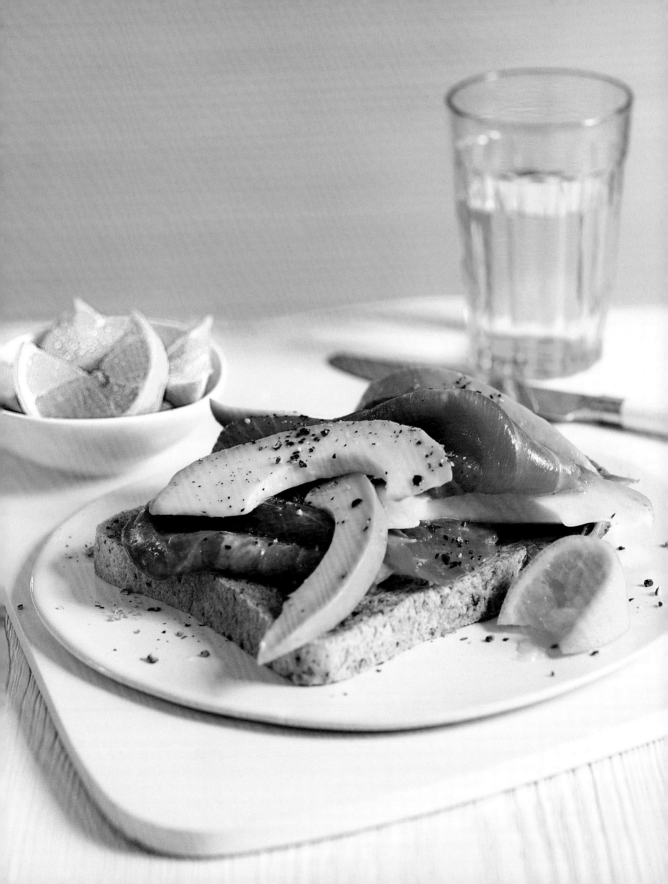

*top tip
You can prepare this awesome source of essential fatty acids beforehand and keep refrigerated in a plastic container

Super Oatmeal

Serves 4

Ingredients

1 apple
3–4 apricots
1¼ cups water
1⅔ cups rolled oats
1¼ cups unsweetened mixed berries, fresh or frozen
10 cardamom pods
2 tablespoons flaxseeds
2 tablespoons hemp seeds
1 teaspoon cinnamon
¼ cup sunflower seeds
¼ cup pumpkin seeds
¼ cup raisins

Method

1. Grate the apple, chop the apricots, and mix in a pan with the water, oats, and half of the berries. Bring to a boil.

2. While the berry mixture is boiling, remove the cardamom from its pods, chop or grind finely, and add to the pan. Boil for 10–15 minutes or until the oats are soft and most of the water has been absorbed or has evaporated, then remove from the heat and set aside to cool a little.

3. Place the flaxseeds and hemp seeds together in a blender and blend thoroughly.

4. Stir the flaxseeds and hemp seeds into the cooled berry mixture, adding plenty of cinnamon.

5. Serve with the remaining fresh berries, sunflower and pumpkin seeds, and raisins.

Perfect Oatmeal

Serves 1

Ingredients

1 cup water/milk/rice milk/almond milk
⅓ cup rolled oats
½ teaspoon ground cinnamon
½ teaspoon orange zest
1 teaspoon toasted sliced almonds

Method

1. Place your liquid of choice in a pan with the oats, ground cinnamon, and orange zest and bring to a boil, then simmer steadily for another 5 minutes, stirring regularly.

2. Serve in a bowl with almonds sprinkled on top.

*serving suggestion
Serve with mixed berries and some greek yogurt

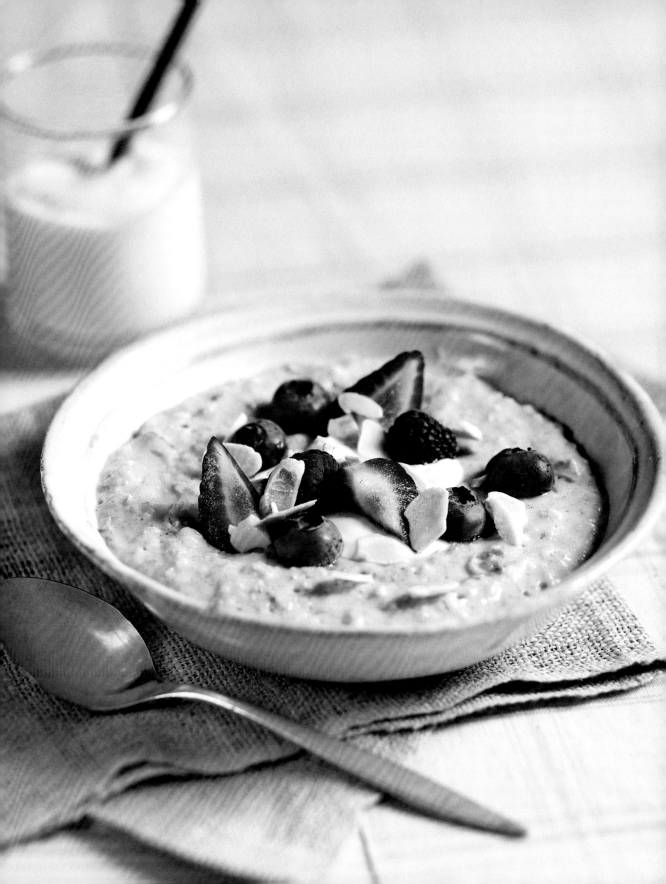

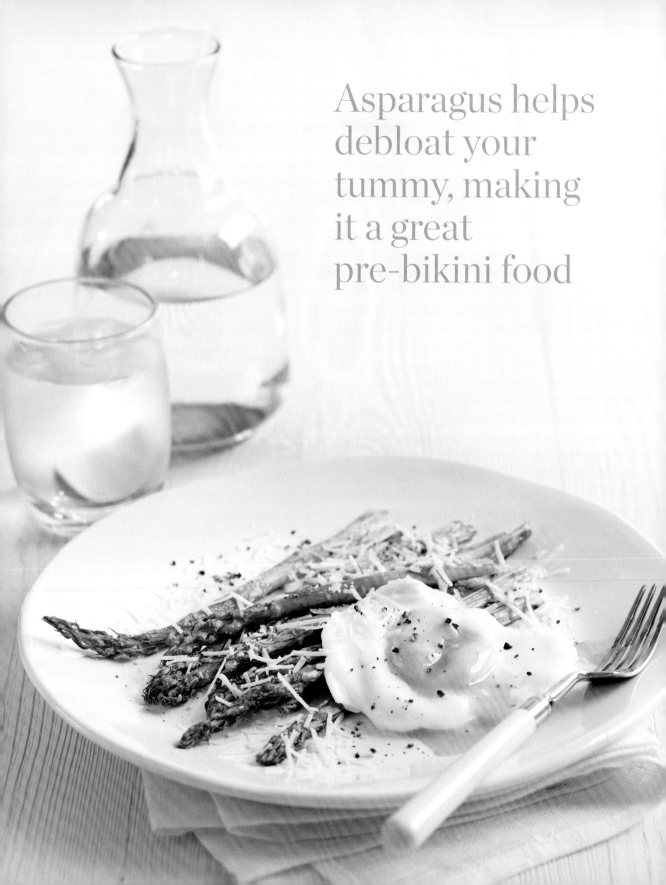

Asparagus helps
debloat your
tummy, making
it a great
pre-bikini food

Poached Eggs with Ham and Spinach

Serves 4

Ingredients
4 organic eggs
4 slices smoked ham
1 cup baby spinach

Method

1. Bring a pan of water to a boil, stir rapidly to create a whirlpool, and crack the first egg into the center; the swirling water should bring the egg together. Repeat with the remaining eggs; 3–4 minutes is sufficient cooking time.

2. Serve each slice of ham with a poached egg on top and spinach on the side.

*remember

Always try to buy organic eggs, or at least free-range, but never battery eggs. Organic eggs have more fat-burning, health-boosting omega-3s, and they taste better too

Hugh Grant's Poached Eggs with Asparagus and Parmesan

Serves 4

Ingredients
2 bunches of asparagus
sea salt and freshly ground black pepper
olive oil, for drizzling
4 fresh organic eggs
Parmesan, for grating

Method

1. Bring a pan of water to a boil and preheat the broiler.

2. Place the asparagus on a baking sheet, season with salt and pepper, and drizzle with olive oil. Broil for approximately 10 minutes, until cooked.

3. Bring a pan of water to a boil, stir rapidly to create a whirlpool, and crack the first egg into the center; the swirling water should bring the egg together. Repeat with the remaining eggs; 3–4 minutes is sufficient cooking time.

4. Serve each egg with asparagus spears and grate a little Parmesan over the top.

Chorizo Frittata

Serves 1

Ingredients
1 teaspoon olive oil
5 slices chorizo
1 scallion, chopped
2 organic eggs
1 tablespoon goat cheese

Method
1. Put the oil in a pan over low heat with the chorizo and scallion and cook for 2 minutes.

2. Meanwhile, whisk the eggs in a bowl, then pour over the ingredients in the pan. Once cooked through, sprinkle the goat cheese over the top and serve.

Goat cheese and Egg White Omelet

Serves 4

Ingredients
3 organic egg yolks
⅓ cup goat cheese
sea salt and freshly ground black pepper
5 organic egg whites
1 teaspoon olive oil

Method
1. In a small bowl, beat the egg yolks, goat cheese, and salt and pepper.

2. In a large bowl or food-processor, beat the egg whites and then fold in the goat cheese mixture.

3. In a frying pan, heat the oil and, once hot, pour in the omelet mixture. Cook for 2 minutes, loosening the sides with an offset spatula, then fold over one half and continue cooking for another 2–3 minutes.

*serving suggestion
Add wilted spinach, roast tomatoes, broiled pancetta, chicken, asparagus, zucchini, chiles, turkey, olives, feta, crab, or shrimp to the omelet before folding in half

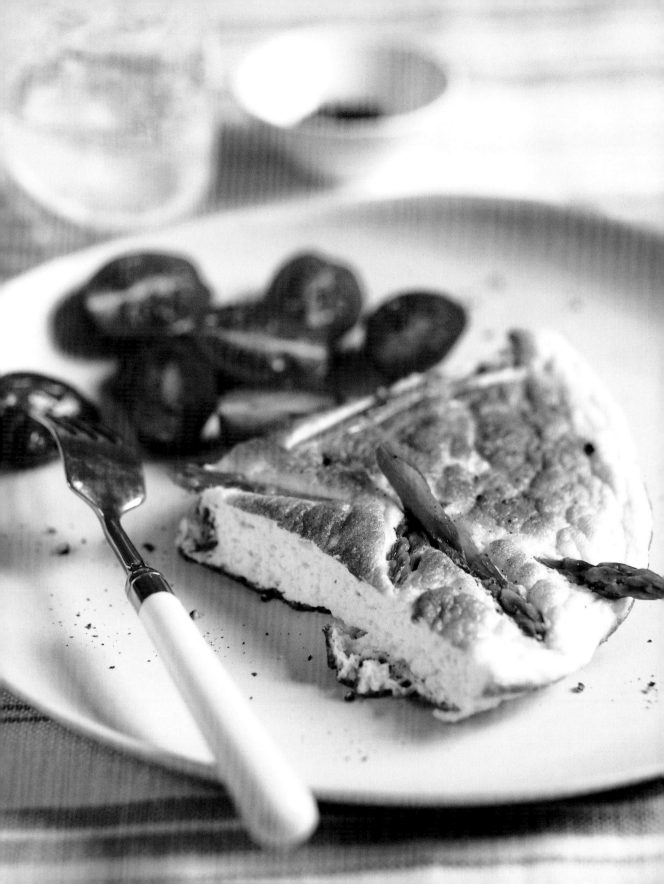

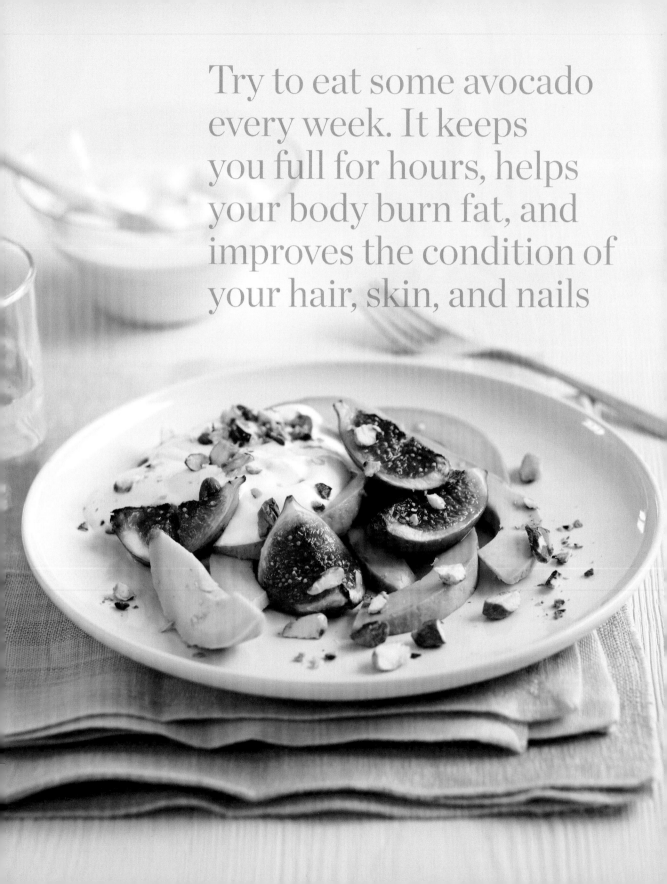

Try to eat some avocado every week. It keeps you full for hours, helps your body burn fat, and improves the condition of your hair, skin, and nails

*note
Don't have eggs every
day. It's good to include
a wide range of protein
in your diet

Broiled Figs with Avocado and Plain Yogurt

Serves 4

Ingredients
4 fresh figs, cut into quarters
2 ripe avocados, halved and sliced
⅔ cup plain yogurt
4 tablespoons shelled pistachios, lightly toasted and chopped

Method
1. Preheat the broiler.

2. Place the figs on a baking sheet and broil until golden.

3. Serve with the sliced avocado, then spoon the yogurt over the top and, finally, sprinkle with the toasted pistachios.

Scrambled Eggs with Smoked Salmon and Roast Asparagus

Serves 4

Ingredients
a bunch of asparagus, trimmed
2 teaspoons olive oil
sea salt and freshly ground black pepper
8 organic eggs
7oz smoked salmon

Method
1. Preheat the oven to 400°F.

2. Lay the asparagus on a sheet of foil, drizzle with 1 teaspoon of the olive oil, and season with salt and pepper. Bring the corners of the foil together to make a sealed parcel and roast in the preheated oven for 8–10 minutes, until the spears are tender.

3. Meanwhile, in a large bowl, beat the eggs with salt and pepper.

4. Heat the remaining olive oil in a frying pan over medium heat, then scramble the eggs using a fork to break them up until cooked to your liking.

5. Serve at once with the smoked salmon and asparagus.

*it's easy
If your mornings are
rushed, you don't
have to cook figs—
just have them fresh
from the fridge

HERE'S MY HANDY "BAD, BETTER & BEST"

BAD	BETTER	BEST
Bad: Breakfast cereal **Why?** Processed and full of salt and sugar	**Better:** Oatmeal made with milk and fresh berries **Why?** Oatmeal is a slow-release carbohydrate with lots of fiber	**Best:** Oatmeal made with organic milk, fresh berries, nuts, and seeds **Why?** The nuts and seeds add healthy fats, which boosts the metabolism and keeps you fuller for longer
Bad: White toast with jam or jelly **Why?** This combination of sugar + sugar will leave you sluggish and hungry well before lunch	**Better:** Whole-grain bread with fresh fruit **Why?** This has more fiber than white bread and jam	**Best:** Dark rye bread with organic nut butter **Why?** This is the perfect blend of slow-release energy carbs and fats
Bad: Fruit juice concentrate **Why?** Sugar with little nutritional value	**Better:** Freshly squeezed juice **Why?** Full of vitamins (but still high in fructose/sugar)	**Best:** A freshly squeezed juice made from cucumber, spinach, and kale **Why?** Sugar-free, alkalizing, nutrient-dense... drink lots of it
Bad: Waffles/pancakes **Why?** Full of sugar and processed flour	**Better:** Gluten-free bread **Why?** No harmful allergens	**Best:** Clean & lean oat pancakes **Why?** A great source of low-GI carbohydrates
Bad: Fried eggs, fried bacon, sausages, and potatoes **Why?** Very high in saturated fat and salt	**Better:** Poached eggs, broiled bacon, and sausages **Why?** Broiling food helps to reduce the saturated fat content of a meal by 25 percent	**Best:** Soft-boiled eggs, broiled organic sausages, and steamed kale or spinach **Why?** Kale is a superfood and organic sausages are rusk- and nitrate-free
Bad: Scrambled eggs and french toast **Why?** Loaded with saturated fat	**Better:** Scrambled eggs with baked beans **Why?** Beans have fiber, but just make sure you get the low-salt version	**Best:** Scrambled eggs with steamed spinach **Why?** High in Vitamin A and iron
Bad: Canned fruit **Why?** Full of sugar (from the syrup) and very low in nutrients	**Better:** Mixed fresh fruit salad **Why?** Contains more vitamins and minerals when fresh	**Best:** Fresh berries with plain yogurt and cinnamon **Why?** A perfect blend of carbs and protein

BREAKFAST GUIDE:

BAD	BETTER	BEST
Bad: Ready-to-eat fruit/crunch yogurts **Why?** Sugar dressed up to be healthy	**Better:** Organic yogurt with fruit compôte **Why?** Organic yogurt is better but the fruit inside the container is still very high in sugar	**Best:** Organic full-fat yogurt with blueberries and mixed nuts **Why?** The perfect blend of protein, fats, carbohydrates, vitamins, and minerals
Bad: Muffin **Why?** Full of sugar, wheat, and flour	**Better:** Gluten-free muffin **Why?** No harmful allergens but still high in sugar	**Best:** Omelet with organic eggs **Why?** Organic eggs are the healthiest source of protein—the gold standard!

*case study

One of my clients used to skip breakfast and power through the morning on coffee. By lunchtime she was starving, so she would eat whatever she could grab quickly that provided quick-release energy, like a sandwich or a bowl of pasta. After she ate it, she would get the inevitable crash in blood-sugar levels (caused by the spike in energy from all those carbs) and would then have to prop her flagging energy levels up with chocolate or something sweet. She just couldn't lose weight because of all those carbs and sugar.

When she came to see me, the first thing I insisted was that she overhaul her breakfast. I still let her have her beloved coffee, but only one or two cups, max. And I only allowed her to have it once she'd eaten breakfast, not before. For breakfast, she had some lovely lean protein, like smoked salmon or eggs, with something green like avocado and a couple of whole-grain crackers. After the first day, she reported fewer sugar cravings, less hunger, and better energy levels all day. By making over her breakfast, the rest of her diet fell into place and she found she could stick to the Clean & Lean regime easily and the weight fell off. But she could only do this once she'd sorted out her bad breakfast habits.

*case study

Another example of a "bad breakfaster" is a friend of mine. She always had sugar-based breakfasts and wondered why she couldn't lose the 5 pounds she wanted to get rid of, and why she was tired all the time (and we all know that tiredness leads to sugar cravings). When she came to me for advice, I asked her what she had for breakfast. She told me: "A croissant or some cereal with skim milk, if I'm being good." Good? Cereal with skim milk is a terrible breakfast, lacking in protein and bursting with sugar. You must, must have protein with your breakfast, if you want to stay full until lunch, and a bit of skim milk just doesn't cut it. As for the croissant, that's another sugar bomb. I told her to ditch the cereal altogether and have some scrambled eggs on rye bread or an omelet filled with greens. If she was busy and didn't have time to make anything, I suggested some full-fat Greek-style yogurt with berries and some whole-grain crackers for a breakfast on the go, or smoked salmon with some avocado. She immediately noticed that her energy levels were better and her sugar cravings were reduced. Thanks to a better breakfast, she stopped snacking on sugar throughout the day and dropped those 5 pounds in less than a month.

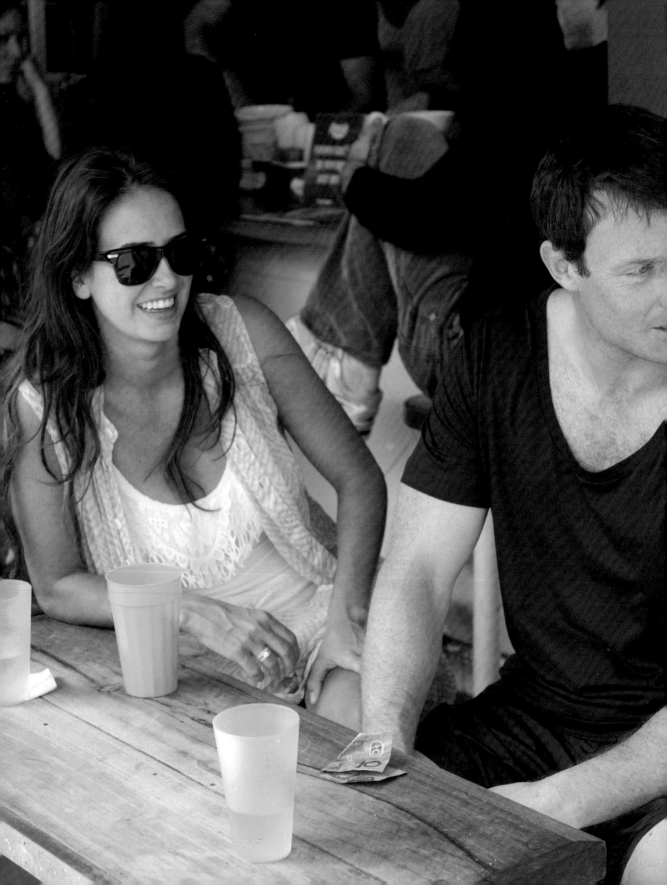

CHAPTER 4

CLEAN AND LEAN LUNCHES

THIS CHAPTER WILL REVEAL:

1. WHY YOU NEED TO DITCH SANDWICHES

2. HOW TO GET THE PERFECT LUNCH, WHEREVER YOU ARE

3. HOW YOU CAN MAKE TASTY LUNCHES IN MINUTES

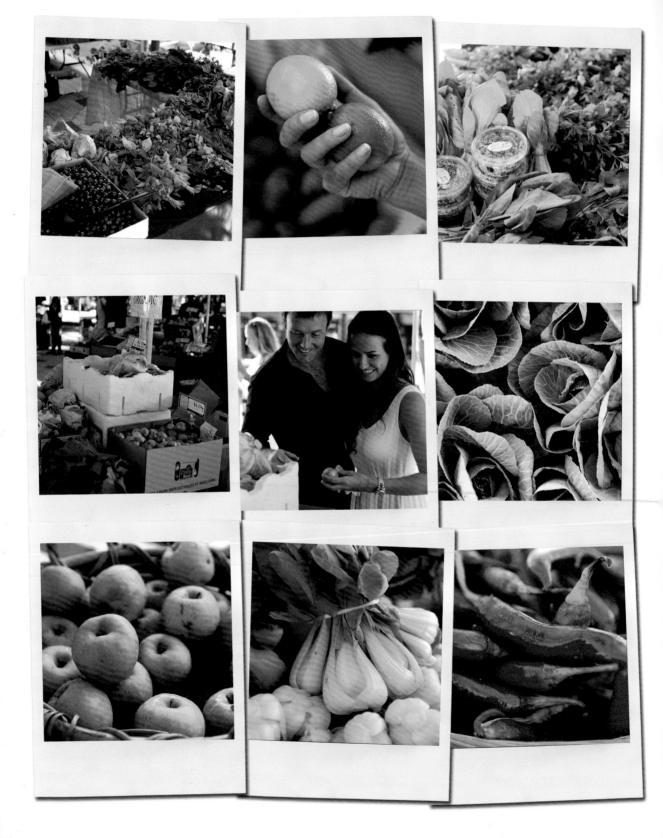

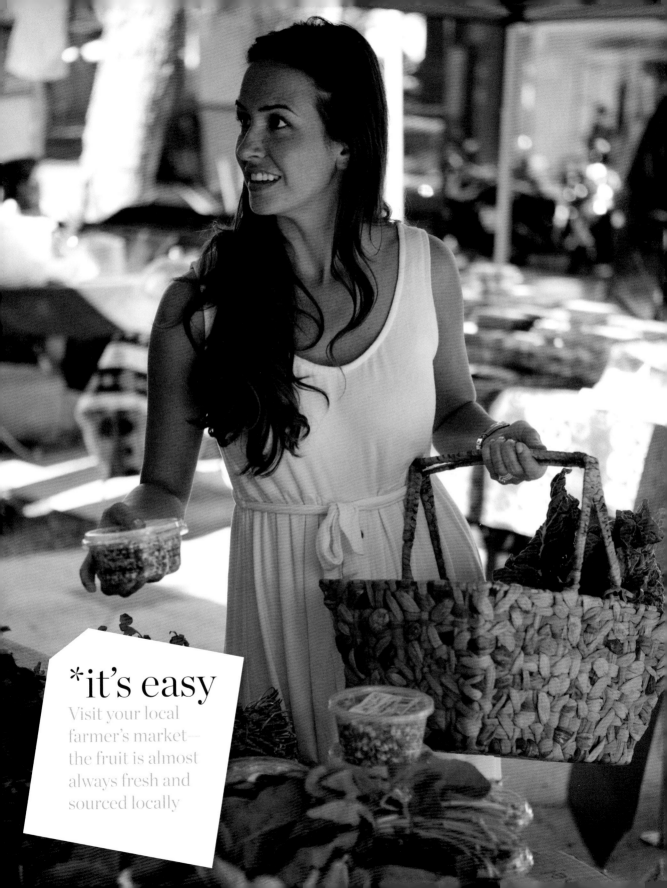

*it's easy

Visit your local farmer's market—the fruit is almost always fresh and sourced locally

Lunch is another important meal to get right. It needs to keep you going for the rest of the day, so if you get it wrong—or skip it altogether—you're likely to binge when it comes to dinner time or you'll spend all afternoon snacking on sugary junk food. This affects your quality of sleep (sugar is a stimulant and chocolate contains caffeine) which slows down fat burning further.

Sadly, for many people, lunch is just something processed, containing barely any protein, grabbed on the go, and eaten quickly, before getting back to work or eaten in front of a computer. Many of my clients have busy jobs in the city or are busy moms, and admit to me that they rarely have time for a proper lunch break. Their lunch usually consists of a pre-packaged sandwich, followed by (yet another) coffee. The result? They're hungry by 3pm and desperate for something sweet to keep them going until dinner time.

A pre-packaged sandwich isn't a good lunch. Take the type you find in the stores—a few slices of (non-organic) chicken, swimming in mayonnaise and squashed between

two slices of processed, salty bread with maybe a few measly limp lettuce leaves and tomato slices. How can that keep you going until dinner? Your lunch needs to contain a decent amount of clean and lean protein—a palm-sized amount, ideally. Tiny bits of meat or fish, the amount you find in your average sandwich, just aren't enough. You also need a large portion of brightly colored vegetables, full of vitamins and minerals that keep you full.

THIS IS WHAT EVERY LUNCH SHOULD CONTAIN:

✳ protein (chicken, fish, eggs, quinoa, tempeh, etc.)
✳ fat (the clean and lean kind, such as half an avocado, a small handful of nuts and seeds, or a good drizzle of olive or coconut oil)
✳ vegetables (include some that are green, such as lettuce, cucumber, and broccoli, and some that are brightly colored, such as tomatoes and peppers).

If I ever have a bad lunch, I feel terrible all afternoon—tired and craving sugar—because I haven't nourished my body properly. So I always try to have a Clean and Lean lunch. My favorite is a salmon and kale salad, which keeps me full and prevents that awful afternoon slump. Wherever I am in the world, I opt for a variation of this—I might swap the salmon for cod, or the kale for green beans or salad.

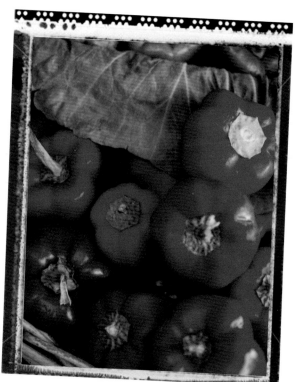

*remember

Take at least a 20 minute break for your lunch and really savor it. If you "stress eat," you don't chew thoroughly and your body won't absorb the nutrients efficiently. Concentrate on your food, not your work, so your body registers you are eating and signals when you are full

COOKING THE CLEAN & LEAN WAY – A QUICK REMINDER

The cleanest ways to cook are:

✷ **Steaming** This is one of the healthiest ways to cook fish, meat, and vegetables. It retains nearly all the nutrients (and flavor) found in food and doesn't add any fat. As the name suggests, the food doesn't come into contact with the water—just the steam that the water lets off. The most common way to do this is to suspend the food over boiling water, using a steamer (this usually has holes in it to allow the steam through).

✷ **Blanching** This is a way of cooking vegetables that keeps them crisp and tender, but also retains lots of the nutrients. You boil them for a short amount of time, so that they're barely cooked but still tender. Then you remove them from the heat, drain, and add them to a bowl of iced water. Wait until they're no longer warm, then quickly reheat them (by boiling, steaming, or broiling for 30 seconds to a minute).

✷ **Broiling** This is a great way to cook meats and fish. Lots of the fat drips away, plus it gives a lovely flavor to your food.

✷ **Baking/roasting** There isn't any real difference between these two. They're both methods of cooking meat, fish, and vegetables using dry heat (your oven), which browns the food's exterior and cooks the middle.

And the worst ways to cook are:

✷ **Frying** Usually, this involves cooking foods with oil in a hot pan. Firstly, the oil soaks into the food and secondly, because that fat is heated up, it becomes less healthy (cold olive oil is far healthier than hot olive oil).

✷ **Boiling** When you boil vegetables they lose many of their health-boosting nutrients. Blanching is OK because you're only boiling them for a short amount of time, but when you just boil your vegetables for a long time, you'll lose too many nutrients.

✷ **Microwaving** It may save you time, but microwaving your food is one of the worst ways to cook. Some studies show it destroys 97 percent of the health-boosting antioxidants found in vegetables.

*it's easy
Save time and don't cook vegetables—you won't lose nutrients that way!

*note
Cold olive oil is much healthier than when it is heated, and it also tastes better too

Clean & Lean Minestrone

Serves 4

Ingredients
¾ cup navy beans
1 onion
1 leek
1 celery rib
1 zucchini
¼ red bell pepper
½ eggplant
7oz spinach
7oz white cabbage
2 tablespoons olive oil
1 garlic clove, finely chopped
1 tablespoon chopped sage
a sprig of thyme
1 small tomato, finely diced
2 cups organic vegetable stock
½ cup tomato juice
a generous pinch of sea salt and freshly
ground black pepper
grated Parmesan, to garnish

Method
1. Soak the beans in water overnight to soften.

2. Dice the onion, leeks, celery, zucchini, red bell pepper, and eggplant, ensuring they're cut the same size.

3. Slice the spinach and cabbage into fine strips.

4. Heat the oil in a large saucepan and add the onions, leeks, celery, and garlic and cook until soft. Add the rest of the vegetables and cook for a few minutes more.

5. Add the sage, thyme, beans, and tomato and cook for another 5 minutes. Add the vegetable stock and tomato juice, bring to a boil, and cook until the vegetables are soft.

6. Lastly, add the cabbage and spinach, season with salt and pepper, and add the grated Parmesan when ready to serve.

*top tip

Soup is great because it hydrates you and keeps you full for hours. Make it in big batches and keep it in the fridge or freezer for a quick and easy meal

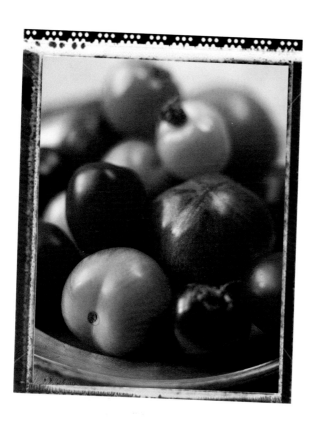

Gazpacho

Serves 2

Ingredients

3 cups fresh tomato juice
4 tablespoons extra virgin olive oil
2 large ripe tomatoes, chopped
1 cucumber, chopped
1 small onion, chopped
1 red bell pepper, seeded and chopped

Method

Place the ingredients in a blender and blend for 1 minute.

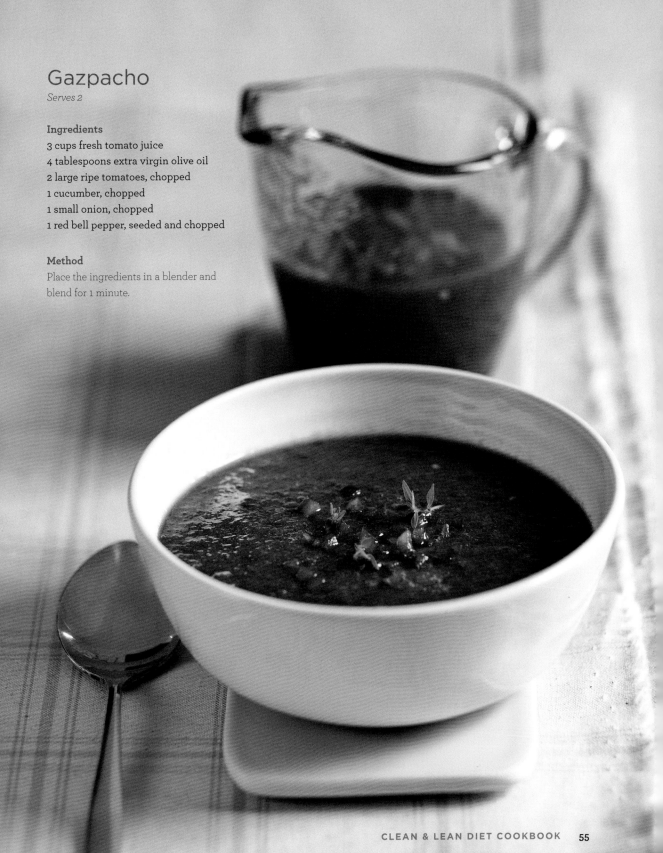

Squash, Ginger, and Sesame Soup

Serves 4

Ingredients

2 tablespoons sesame oil
1 onion, chopped
2 celery ribs, sliced
2 carrots, peeled and chopped
2 garlic cloves, chopped
1 x 2in piece of fresh ginger, peeled and finely chopped
a bunch of cilantro, roots and leaves separated and chopped
1 butternut or acorn squash, peeled and cut into chunks
1 quart organic vegetable or chicken stock
sea salt and freshly ground black pepper
2 tablespoons sesame seeds, lightly toasted

Method

1. Heat the oil in a large pan over medium heat, then add the onion, celery, carrots, garlic, ginger, and cilantro roots and cook for 10 minutes.

2. Add the squash and cook for another 10 minutes, or until it begins to soften.

3. Add the stock and salt and pepper, bring to a boil, and simmer for roughly 20-25 minutes, until the squash is cooked.

4. Place the soup in a blender and pulse until smooth. Adjust the seasoning and serve topped with the toasted sesame seeds.

Spinach, Pea, and Tarragon Soup

Serves 4

Ingredients

2 tablespoons olive oil
1 onion, chopped
1 leek, thinly sliced
2 garlic cloves, chopped
a bunch of tarragon
8oz baby spinach
1 quart organic vegetable or chicken stock
sea salt and freshly ground black pepper
2¾ cups petit pois
juice of ½ lemon
extra virgin olive oil, for drizzling

Method

1. In a large pan, heat the oil and gently cook the onion, leek, and garlic until softened, approximately 10 minutes.

2. Add the tarragon and spinach, and once the leaves are wilted, add the stock and salt and pepper. Bring to a boil and add half the peas. Cook for another 5 minutes, then remove from the heat.

3. Place the soup in a blender and pulse until smooth, then add the lemon juice and the remaining peas. Adjust the seasoning if necessary before serving with a drizzle of extra virgin olive oil.

Fava Bean Dip

Serves 4

Ingredients

2⅔ cups fava beans, fresh or frozen,
shelled weight
¾ cup plain organic yogurt
juice of 1 lemon
1 garlic clove, crushed
sea salt and freshly ground black pepper
4 tablespoons extra virgin olive oil
a small bunch of mint, very finely chopped
1 tablespoon tahini paste

Method

1. Blanch the beans in a pan of boiling salted
water for 4 minutes. Drain and run under
cold water.

2. Place the beans in a blender with all the
other ingredients and process until smooth.
Taste for seasoning and adjust if necessary.

Spinach and Artichoke Dip

Serves 4

Ingredients

a large handful of spinach
⅓ cup canned artichoke hearts
¼ cup grated Parmesan
1 garlic clove
squeeze of lemon juice
½ cup sour cream
dill and parsley (about 10g
each), to taste

Method

1. Preheat the oven to 350°F.

2. Place all the ingredients in a
blender and blend for approximately
30 seconds. Pour into an ovenproof
dish and bake in the preheated
oven for 20 minutes.

Guacamole

Serves 4

Ingredients

2 ripe avocados
1 medium tomato
juice of ½ lemon
½ red onion
sea salt, to taste

Method

Place all the ingredients in a
blender and pulse for 20 seconds
or until desired consistency
is reached.

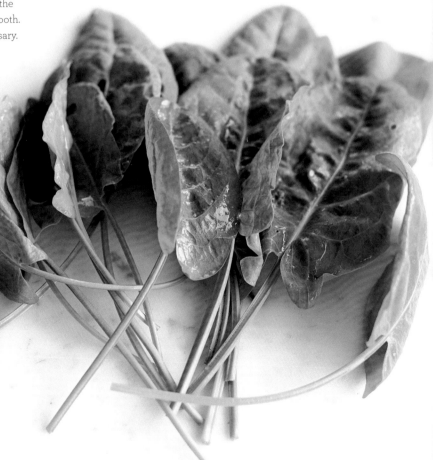

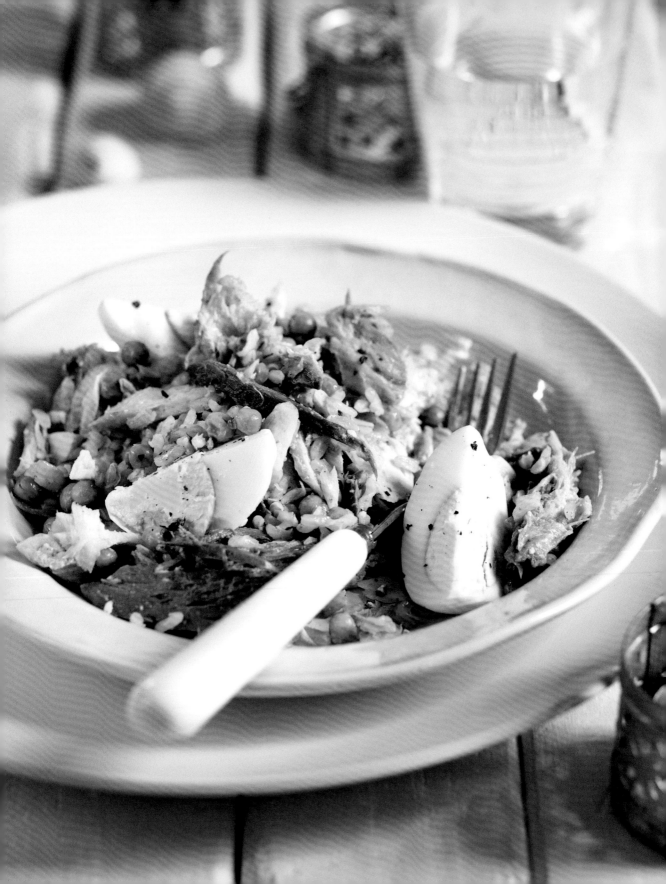

Mackerel Kedgeree

Serves 4

Ingredients

1 tablespoon olive oil
1 onion, finely chopped
1 teaspoon ground coriander
1 teaspoon curry powder
1½ cups brown rice, cooked and drained
⅔ cup peas
4 naturally smoked mackerel fillets,
flesh flaked off the bone
sea salt and freshly ground black pepper
2 hard-boiled organic eggs, peeled and
quartered, to garnish

Method

1. In a large frying pan, heat the oil and gently cook the onion until soft and translucent.

2. Add the ground coriander and curry powder and continue cooking for another 2-3 minutes. Stir in the rice, the peas, and the fish. Season with salt and pepper and cook over low heat, stirring continuously.

3. Serve garnished with the eggs.

This is a tasty favorite—it takes about 3 minutes and is full of nutrients and minerals. Couldn't be easier or quicker! It's good for a snack any time of day and great for kids as well; and you can throw in any leftovers you may have in the fridge as well to really mix it up
Elle Macpherson

Elle's Quick Scrambled Eggs

Serves 1

Ingredients

2 organic eggs
generous pinch of sea salt and freshly
ground black pepper
splash of milk
½ tablespoon unsalted butter
1 scallion
a pinch of red pepper flakes

Method

1. Break the eggs into a bowl, season, and whisk together with a splash of milk.

2. Heat the butter in a saucepan until it is melted and then add the egg mixture, stirring all the time until they are scrambled and cooked to your liking.

3. Turn the eggs onto a plate, scatter the scallions over the top, and add a sprinkling of red pepper flakes to taste.

*top tip

I've had this salad several times and it's yummy. It's great because it's bursting with flavor and so complete—meaning it contains good fat from the avocado, oil, goat cheese, and seeds plus vitamins from the kale and other vegetables. Kale is also one of the most alkaline foods, which means it reduces inflammation in the body and boosts your immune system

Elle's Kale and Goat Cheese Salad

Serves 2

Ingredients

4 large handfuls of kale
a sprinkle of goat cheese
a sprinkle of sunflower and pumpkin seeds
½ avocado
2 red radishes, thinly sliced
sea salt and freshly ground black pepper, to taste
juice of ½ lemon
2 tablespoons olive oil

Method

Put the kale, goat cheese, seeds, avocado, and radishes in a bowl and mix. Season to taste, then dress with the lemon juice and olive oil.

Scallion, Watercress, and Tarragon Frittata

Serves 4

Ingredients

1½ tablespoons olive oil
a bunch of scallions, trimmed and sliced, using the majority of the green leaves
2 garlic cloves, crushed
a bunch of tarragon
a bunch of watercress, leaves and thin stems picked off
8 organic eggs
sea salt and freshly ground black pepper
½ tablespoon olive oil

Method

1. In a small frying pan, heat the oil over medium heat and cook the scallions, garlic, and tarragon until softened. Add the watercress and continue cooking until wilted.

2. In a mixing bowl, whisk the eggs and add the salt and pepper. Add the scallion mix and combine well.

3. In a small frying pan, heat the olive oil and add the frittata mix. Over medium-low heat, cook the frittata, pulling in the edges with a spatula. Meanwhile, preheat the broiler. After roughly 8 minutes, once the frittata is cooked on the bottom, place the pan under the broiler and cook for another 5–8 minutes, until golden and cooked.

4. Enjoy with a green salad.

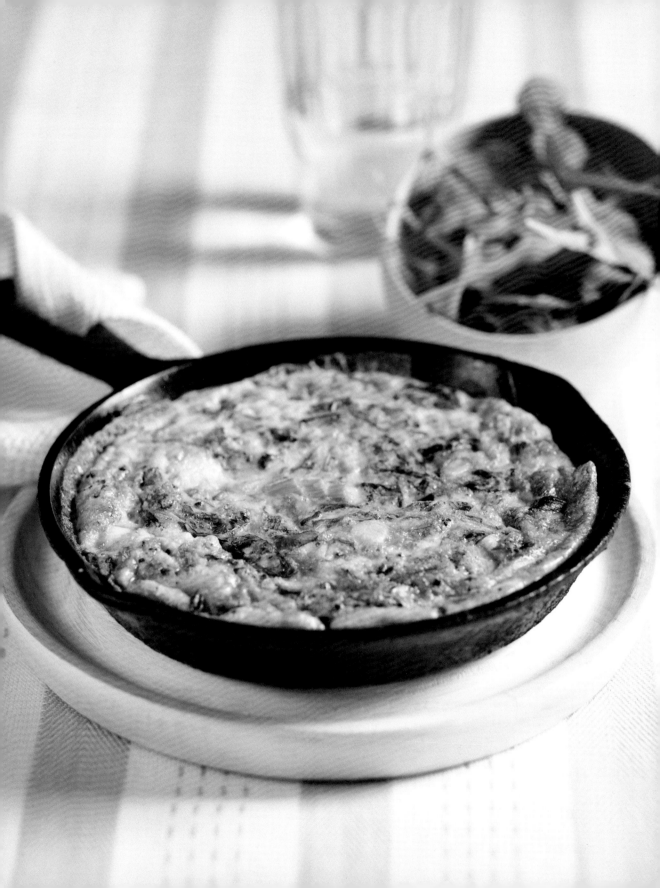

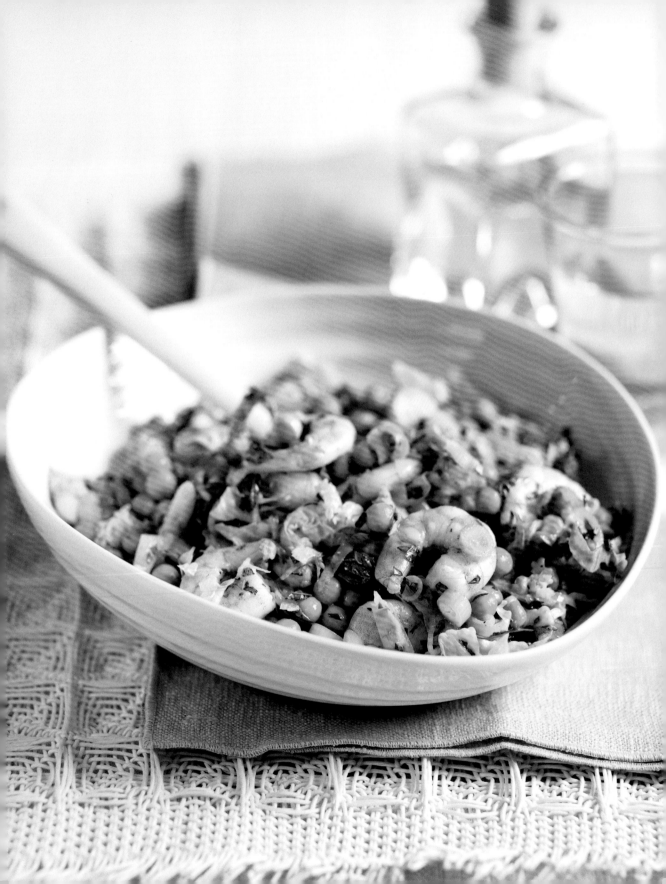

Pea, Shrimp, and Tarragon Salad

Serves 4

Ingredients
9oz cooked shrimp
1½ cups peas, cooked
4 scallions, finely chopped
1 baby gem lettuce, shredded finely
a small bunch of tarragon, finely chopped
a small bunch of mint, finely chopped

For the dressing
2 tablespoons extra virgin olive oil
1 teaspoon white wine or tarragon vinegar
1 teaspoon Dijon mustard
sea salt and freshly ground black pepper

Method
1. In a large salad bowl, toss together the shrimp, peas, scallions, lettuce, and herbs.

2. For the dressing, whisk the remaining ingredients and pour over the salad.

3. Toss the salad again before serving.

*top tip
Shrimp is a fantastic choice of protein—it is low in fat, keeps you full, and is super easy and versatile to cook with

*top tip
This is a fantastic meal. The ingredients in it are nourishing and energizing and the garlic will protect your heart

Zoe Kravitz's Big Bowl of Love

Serves 1

Ingredients
2 tablespoons olive oil
6 stems purple-sprouting broccoli
2 large handfuls of baby spinach
1 garlic clove, crushed
1 mackerel or trout fillet
a small dab of harissa paste
⅓ cup cooked brown rice
a handful of bean sprouts

Method
1. Preheat the broiler.

2. Heat the olive oil in a sauté pan and cook the broccoli for 2 minutes, then add the spinach and crushed garlic, stirring until it smells amazing and softens slightly.

3. Prepare the fish with either a dab of harissa paste or a sprinkle of chile powder and lemon juice, and broil for 2–3 minutes on each side.

4. Toss all the vegetables together in a large bowl and serve with the fish, rice, and bean sprouts.

Delicious Beluga Salad

Serves 4

Ingredients

1 x 7oz can beluga lentils (available in specialty stores)
water (enough to cover the lentils by 1in)
1½ cups small sweet tomatoes, halved
1 bay leaf
a large bunch of parsley, chopped and stems reserved
a large bunch of cilantro, chopped and stems reserved
1 large red onion, finely chopped
½ garlic clove, finely chopped
sea salt and freshly ground black pepper
juice of 3–4 limes
splash of balsamic vinegar
½ red, green, and yellow bell peppers, finely chopped
2 ripe avocados, diced
4 tablespoons olive oil
7oz mixed salad leaves and baby spinach

Method

1. Rinse and pick out any dirt from the lentils. Place the lentils in a saucepan with the water, one third of the tomatoes, a bay leaf, and the stems from the parsley and cilantro. Don't worry about how much water you put in to start with, just add more as needed. Bring to a boil, then reduce to a simmer. (You need all the water to be absorbed, so the lentils are soft, but not too wet.)

2. While the lentils are boiling (30–35 minutes), place the red onion and garlic in a bowl. Add the salt and pepper, lime juice, and balsamic vinegar. Let the onion marinate in the liquid while the lentils are boiling.

3. When the lentils are done and seasoned, let them cool until they are lukewarm, then remove the bay leaf and add the lentils to the red onion and garlic.

4. Add the bell peppers, the chopped herbs, and the remaining tomatoes and avocados. Season with some olive oil, freshly ground black pepper and salt, and maybe some more lime juice. The idea is to get a bit of warmth from the ground black pepper and acidity from the lime and to combine the freshness of the cilantro with the buttery taste of ripe avocado.

5. Serve on a bed of mixed salad leaves and baby spinach.

*top tip

This is a great dish for vegans. Always add some (healthy) fat to your salads because it helps your body absorb the nutrients from the vegetables more efficiently. Add a drizzle of oil, some avocado, or a sprinkling of nuts

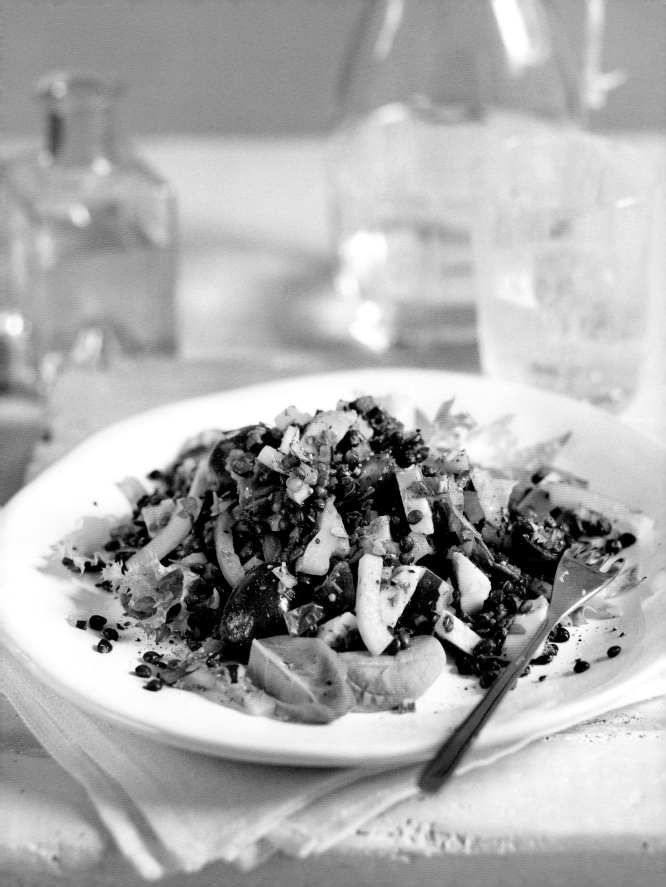

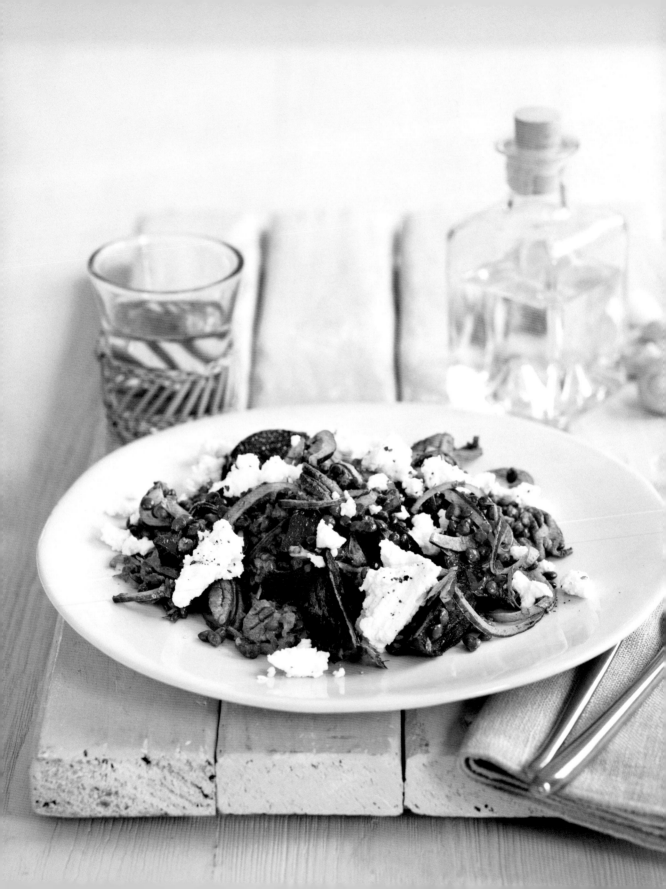

Lentils, Pecan, and Roasted Beet Salad with Goat Cheese

Serves 4

Ingredients

4 large raw beets, scrubbed and
peeled if skin is thick
4 garlic cloves
1 cup puy lentils
1 red onion, finely sliced
1 tablespoon flaxseed oil
1 teaspoon Dijon mustard
1 teaspoon red wine vinegar
sea salt and freshly ground black pepper
a small bunch of parsley
1 cup pecans, toasted and roughly chopped
⅓ cup goat cheese

Method

1. Preheat the oven to 400°F.

2. Wrap the beets together with a garlic clove in foil and roast in the oven for approximately 45 minutes or until tender. Let cool and then peel and cut into small wedges.

3. Meanwhile, place the lentils in a pan and cover with cold water. Bring to a boil and simmer for approximately 15–20 minutes until cooked, but with bite. Drain and toss with the red onions and beets.

4. Whisk together the oil, mustard, vinegar, and salt and pepper. Pour the mixture over the lentils and mix in the parsley. Add the pecans and serve topped with goat cheese.

Quiche with Brown Rice Crust

Serves 4

Ingredients
For the brown rice crust
1½ cups cooked brown rice
1 organic egg white

For the filling
vegetables of your choice, e.g. broccoli, bell peppers, spinach
3 large organic eggs
½ cup Cheddar cheese, shredded
¾ cup rice milk
herbs of your choice, e.g. basil, parsley

Method

1. Preheat the oven to 350°F. Lightly oil an 8-inch deep-dish pie plate.

2. To make the crust, mix the ingredients by hand, then press into the base of the pie plate with the back of a spoon to make compact.

3. Place in the preheated oven and bake for 10 minutes. Remove from the oven and turn the heat up to 400°F.

4. Place your chosen vegetables on the bottom of the cooked brown rice crust.

5. Mix the remaining filling ingredients in a blender for 30 seconds, then pour over the vegetables and bake for 40 minutes.

*serving suggestion

This goes well with turkey breast or any other clean and lean protein like chicken or white fish

Hugh Grant's Cold Lamb Salad

Serves 4

4 slices cold, pre-cooked lamb
4 large tomatoes, sliced
9oz mozzarella, sliced
pinch of sea salt and freshly ground
black pepper
olive oil, for drizzling

Method
Simply arrange the ingredients on a plate,
season with a twist of pepper, and drizzle
with olive oil. Enjoy!

*When my good friend and
mentor, James Duigan told me
he was writing another bestseller,
I couldn't stop giggling with
excitement. I read his recipes
every night and I already feel
thinner. James is very handsome.*
Hugh Grant

Red and Yellow Salad with Seared Mackerel

Serves 4

Ingredients
1 yellow bell pepper, finely sliced
1 pint cherry tomatoes, quartered
2 carrots, peeled and grated
a bunch of cilantro, leaves picked
off stems
2 tablespoon pumpkin seeds, lightly
toasted
1 tablespoon flaxseed oil
juice of ½ lemon
sea salt and freshly ground black pepper
4 mackerel fillets
olive oil, for drizzling

Method
1. Mix together the bell pepper, tomatoes,
carrots, cilantro, and pumpkin seeds, then
dress with the flaxseed oil, lemon juice, and
salt and pepper.

2. Score the skin of the mackerel fillets and
season both sides with salt and pepper.

3. Heat a heavy-bottomed frying pan and
drizzle the skin of the fish with olive oil. Sear
skin-side down first for 2–3 minutes, then flip
and repeat on the flesh side.

4. Serve the mackerel with the salad.

Green Super Salad
Serves 4

Ingredients
1 cup green beans, trimmed
a bunch of asparagus, trimmed
3½oz baby spinach
a small bunch of arugula
½ cucumber, halved, seeded, and sliced
¾ cup frozen peas, defrosted
2 tablespoons pine nuts, lightly toasted

For the dressing
a small bunch of basil, finely chopped
a small bunch of tarragon, finely chopped
3 tablespoons extra virgin olive oil
2 teaspoons white wine vinegar
1 teaspoon Dijon mustard
sea salt and freshly ground black pepper

Method
1. Blanch the green beans and asparagus quickly in a pan of boiling salted water until tender with a little bite. Drain and run under cold water to cool and prevent them from cooking any further. Cut the tips off the asparagus and set aside.

2. In a large salad bowl, toss together the spinach, arugula, and cucumber. Scatter with the peas, asparagus stalks, and green beans, then sprinkle with the pine nuts and the reserved asparagus tips.

3. To make the dressing, whisk together the herbs, olive oil, vinegar, mustard, and salt and pepper. Pour over the salad and enjoy!

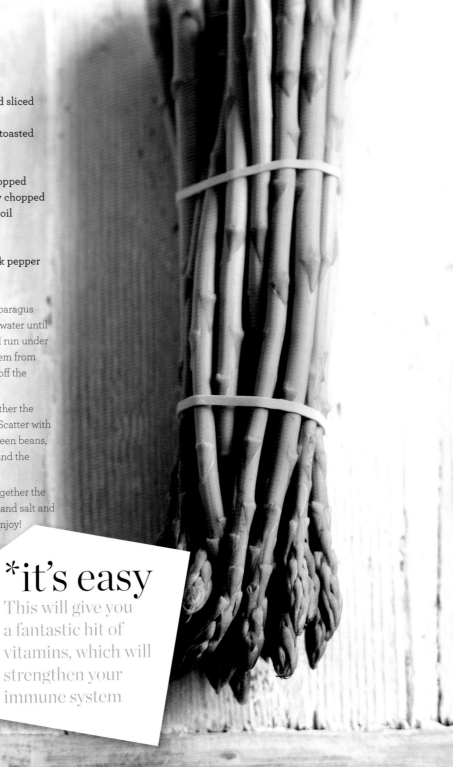

*it's easy
This will give you a fantastic hit of vitamins, which will strengthen your immune system

Crunchy Cambodian-Style Beef Salad

Serves 4

Ingredients
1lb 2oz beef tenderloin
1 teaspoon olive oil
sea salt and freshly ground black pepper

For the salad
2 celery ribs, cut into thin strips
½ cucumber peeled, seeded, and cut into thin strips
raw/green mango cut into thin strips, optional (a handful of pomegranate works well with beef too when raw/green mango is not available)
a handful of bean sprouts
sea salt and freshly ground black pepper
lime juice, to taste
1 teaspoon olive oil

To serve
1 red onion, diced
a handful of crushed cashews, to serve

For the dressing
2 garlic cloves, crushed
1 red chile
a bunch of cilantro
juice of 2 limes
2 teaspoons finely chopped fresh ginger
2 tablespoons chicken stock
sea salt and freshly ground black pepper, to taste

Method

1. Heat a grill pan until very hot.

2. Rub the beef tenderloin with the olive oil and a small pinch of salt and pepper and grill until medium-rare, about 2–3 minutes on each side. Let stand while you prepare the salad.

3. In a large bowl, toss all the salad ingredients together with the salt, pepper, lime juice, and olive oil. Transfer to a serving plate in a crunchy, neat mound.

4. Thinly slice the beef and lay on top of the salad mound. Top with the red onion and crushed cashews.

5. To make the dressing, mix the garlic and chile to a paste then mix in the remaining ingredients. Pour over the meat and salad and serve.

*serving suggestion
Chicken is also delicious with this salad. Poach an organic skinless chicken breast in water with a tablespoon of Chinese sherry, a sprinkle of palm sugar, and a pod of star anise, then let cool while you prepare the salad

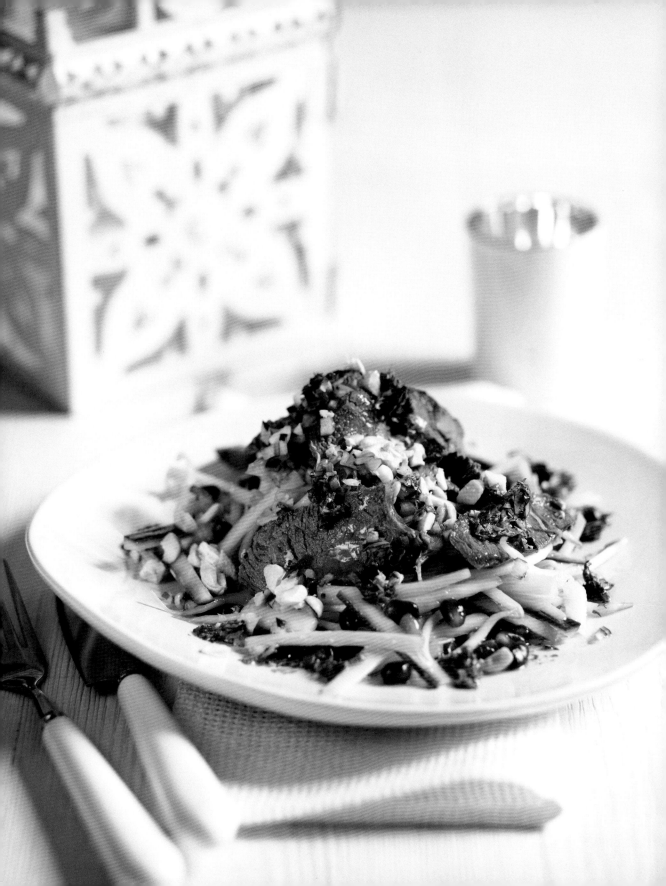

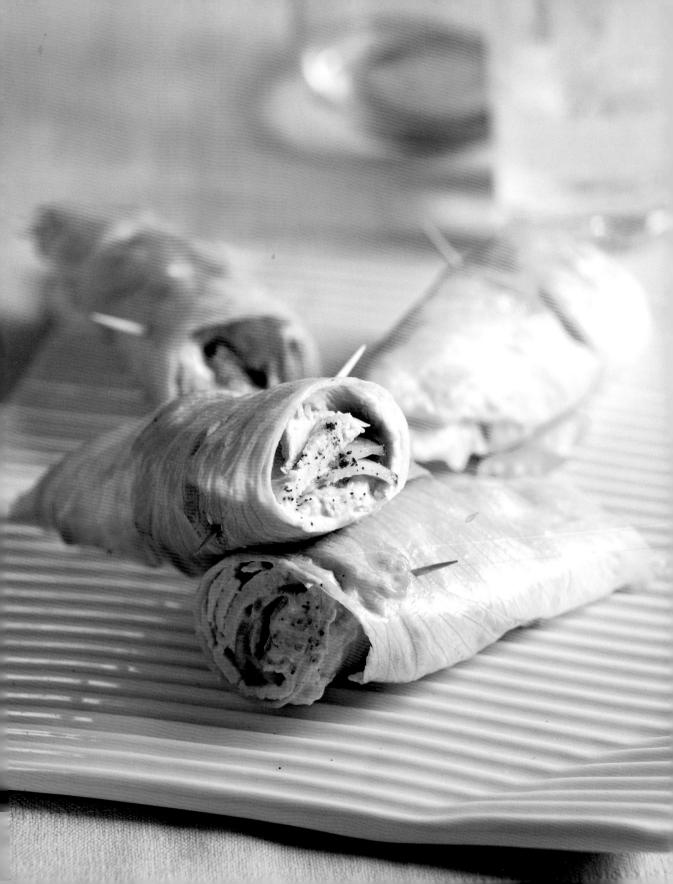

Ultimate Clean & Lean Lettuce Wrap

Serves 4

Ingredients

4 leaves iceberg lettuce
4 slices roast turkey
½ cucumber, sliced
1 cup hummus
sprinkle of paprika

Method

Top a lettuce leaf with a slice of turkey, cucumber, hummus, and paprika, then, as if it were a sandwich, wrap it up with another piece of lettuce. Repeat with the remaining ingredients.

*it's easy

A lettuce wrap makes for a quick and easy packed lunch for work and the variety is endless!

I love the Clean & Lean approach to diet and life—it's so simple and yet so effective. Once I had James' Clean & Lean mantra in my head, I found it easy to stay in shape with the right food, supplements, and lifestyle choices, although I have to say my favorite part is the yummy shakes he makes.
Rosie Huntington-Whiteley

*serving suggestion

This can be done with a variety of ingredients, such as tomatoes, avocados, or bell peppers, as well as salmon, chicken, lamb, or shrimp. White cheeses, herbs, garlic, lemon juice, paprika, turmeric, and oregano all work too. Whatever you have in your fridge!

Zucchini and Lamb Skewers

Serves 4

Ingredients

14oz lean lamb, diced into large chunks
2 zucchini, cut into thick rounds
2 red onions, cut into quarters
2 tablespoons olive oil
1 garlic clove, crushed
sea salt and freshly ground black pepper
4 wooden skewers soaked in water for
30 minutes
a bunch of arugula
a small bunch of basil, leaves removed
from stems
1⅔ cups feta cheese
juice of 1 lemon
extra virgin olive oil, for drizzling

Method

1. Preheat the broiler.

2. Toss the lamb pieces, zucchini, and red onions in the olive oil, crushed garlic, salt, and pepper. Thread onto the prepared skewers, alternating between the lamb, zucchini, and red onions. Place under the preheated broiler for roughly 7–10 minutes before turning and repeating. Check the lamb to ensure it's cooked to your liking.

3. Toss together the arugula, basil, and feta and dress with lemon juice and olive oil and serve with the skewers.

Chicken Skewers

Serves 4

Ingredients

4 chicken breasts, cut into chunks
juice of 2 lemons
1 lemongrass stalk, broken into pieces
1 red chile, chopped
a bunch of cilantro, chopped (optional)
20 cherry tomatoes
sea salt and freshly ground black pepper,
to taste
4 wooden skewers, soaked for 30 minutes
4 coconut leaves or parchment paper

Method

1. Preheat the oven to 400°F.

2. Place the chicken, lemon juice, lemongrass, chile, and cilantro, if using, in a bowl and mix well. Cover and leave in the fridge to infuse for 30 minutes–2 hours.

3. Thread the chicken and the tomatoes onto the skewers, evenly distributed between them.

4. Place the skewers on the coconut leaves or parchment paper and make into little parcels—folding the leaves around and tying with kitchen string. Place on a baking sheet and cook in the preheated oven for 16–20 minutes.

5. Serve with a fresh green salad and some guacamole (see recipe on p. 57).

*serving suggestion

These skewers taste great on an outdoor grill, which adds a lovely smoky flavor and avoids the need for other seasoning and condiments

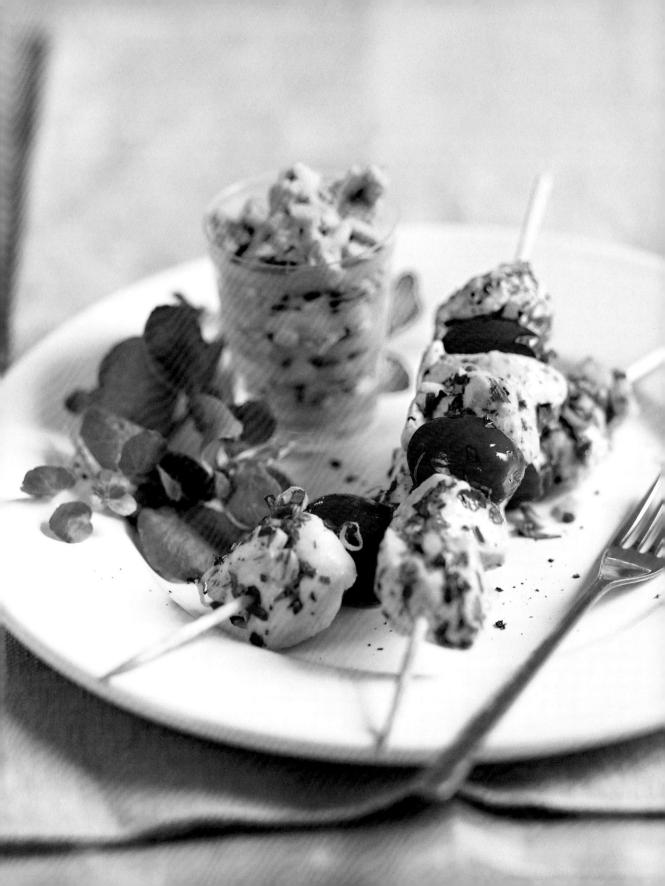

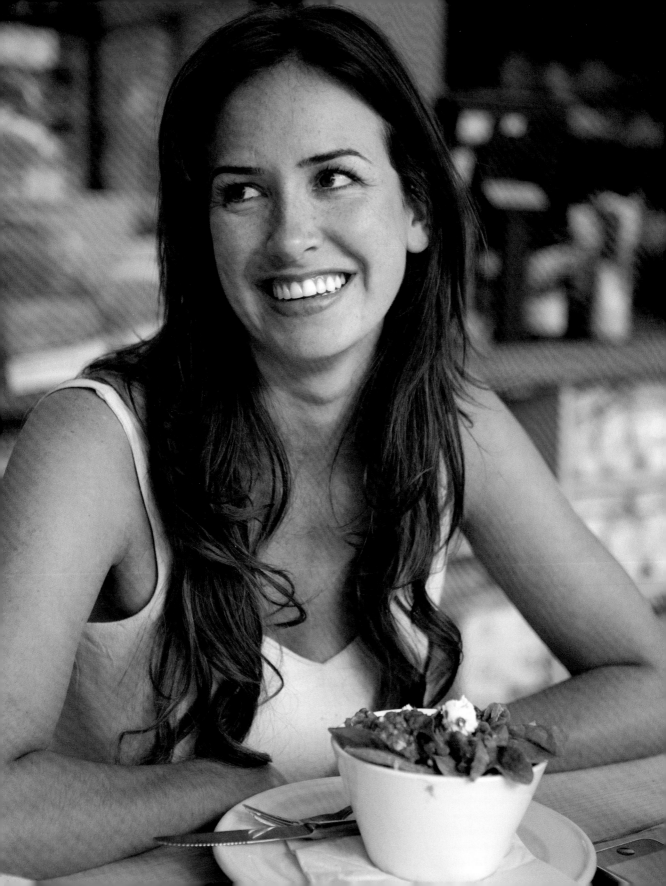

QUICK TIPS FOR LUNCHES ON THE GO

You won't always have time to make your lunch, especially if you work in an office. So here are my tips for lunches to go.

If you go to a sandwich bar...

✻ Go for a wrap instead of bread—it contains fewer carbohydrates than two slices of bread and will leave you less bloated.

✻ Get it with as much protein as possible— tuna, chicken, lamb, etc., and ask for extra, if necessary. Most places will give you a tiny sliver of chicken that won't keep you full and will cause you to snack.

✻ Don't drink your calories. Just stick to water and avoid sodas or juice, which are full of sugars. And don't drink during your lunch; instead, make sure you're hydrated by sipping water throughout the morning.

If you make your own lunch...

✻ Bring leftover cold proteins. Even in winter, you don't need a hot lunch, so change your mindset on that one. I always have leftover proteins at work—they are super healthy, super easy to make, and don't require any preparation. I love salmon, but you could also try chicken, beef, shrimp, or even a couple of hard-boiled eggs.

✻ Have your leftovers with salad or some pre-cooked vegetables (don't overcook so they retain some crunch).

✻ Think outside the box. Forget what you think a proper lunch "should" be and just take a selection of healthy foods to eat. For example, if all you have in your cupboards are whole-grain crackers, some nuts, an apple, and leftover chicken, have those for your lunch. It will fill you up, takes no time, and will keep you nice and slim.

If you go to a pizzeria...

✻ This is a tough one, so all I can say here is to aim for damage control. If you go to a place that serves pasta as well, opt for this with a meatball topping or, even better, broiled fish with a side salad.

✻ If you must have pizza, ask for extra protein (chicken or shrimp) and order a side salad or some vegetables as well.

If you go to a salad bar

✻ Load up on brightly colored vegetables as the reds, oranges, and yellows are a result of the nutrients in them. An orange bell pepper, for example, is a sign of vitamin A.

✻ Avoid cheese, croutons, raisins, pasta, and creamy dressings.

✻ Add good fat to your salad, with avocado, olive oil (the best dressing to go for at a salad bar), or oily fish, like salmon.

If you go for sushi...

✻ This is a really easy one—go for sashimi (raw fish) and edamame beans and salad.

✻ Avoid dishes with rice, where possible. Sushi restaurants often use rice wine and sugar to bind their rice.

*remember

You should have a palm-sized amount of protein with your lunch. Any less and you'll be hungry in the afternoon

CLEAN & LEAN OILS

* Extra virgin olive oil
* Macadamia nut oil
* Avocado oil
* Coconut oil
* Sesame oil

CLEAN & LEAN NUTS AND SEEDS

* Almonds
* Pecans
* Walnuts
* Brazil nuts
* Pistachios
* Macadamia nuts
* Cashews
* Chestnuts
* Peanuts
* Sunflower seeds
* Sesame seeds
* Pumpkin seeds
* Flax seeds (ground only)

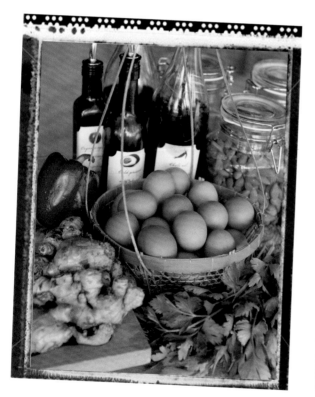

WHY WE LOVE COCONUT OIL

The health benefits of coconut oil are phenomenal and it's fast becoming a superfood thanks to its A-list following (models swear by it!). Here's why you need to go out and buy some this week...It helps with weight loss, it can ease digestive problems such as bloating, strengthen your immunity, and keep your cholesterol levels healthy, and it also makes your hair shiny and your skin glow.

Many models include coconut oil in their diet because it helps the body to metabolize fat, meaning you burn more calories. You can cook with it (it's one of the few oils that retain its health benefits when heated, unlike olive oil), drizzle it cold on salad, have a teaspoon of it in herbal tea, or pour it over just about anything, from poached eggs to grilled vegetables. I would suggest you have around 4 teaspoons a day. It tastes absolutely delicious—very nutty and fresh—and you can buy it in most health stores and some supermarkets.

You can apply coconut oil directly onto your skin as it will be absorbed and can soothe dry skin conditions. You can also apply it directly on the hair. Use it like a hair mask, leaving for a few minutes to soak in, and then rinse.

FOODS TO AVOID
* Canned foods (with added sugar + preservatives)
* White bread, pasta, and rice
* Processed meats
* Breakfast cereals
* Frozen meals
* Frozen potatoes, fries, etc.
* Packages of dried pasta
* Packaged cakes, cookies, muffins
* Chocolate, sweets, and chips

"BAD, BETTER & BEST" LUNCH GUIDE:

BAD	BETTER	BEST
Bad: Cheeseburger **Why?** Non-organic meat is loaded with hormones and the bun is full of sugar and salt	**Better:** Burger (no bun) with salad **Why?** Make sure the salad is colorful, so full of antioxidants, and add avocado for some healthy fats	**Best:** Clean & Lean lettuce wrap with lean meat or cheese **Why?** The superhero of quick, easy lunches—a perfect balance of protein, carbs, and good fat
Bad: Store-bought white bread club sandwich **Why?** Full of unhealthy fats, processed meats, and salt	**Better:** Rye bread sandwich with mustard and protein **Why?** Mustard helps speed up your metabolism	**Best:** Ditch the bread—just eat the sandwich filling **Why?** Choose fillings like chicken, turkey, beef, and tuna and serve with heaps of nutritious, colorful salad
Bad: Sushi rolls with white rice **Why?** Contains very little of nutritional value	**Better:** Sushi rolls with brown rice **Why?** Brown rice has more fiber than white rice and is great for digestion	**Best** Sashimi with seaweed salad **Why?** Seaweed is a powerful antioxidant and helps rid the body of toxins
Bad: Caesar salad **Why?** Most salad dressings are full of unhealthy fats and packed with sugar and salt	**Better:** Caesar salad with grilled chicken but no croutons, and a splash of lemon juice and olive oil **Why?** Salads dressed like this are much healthier and the protein keeps you feel fuller for longer	**Best:** Clean & Lean super salad **Why?** A salad with organic protein, seeds, and nuts is the perfect lunch
Bad: Fish and chips **Why?** Fried foods are loaded with unhealthy trans fats	**Better:** Fried fish with no batter and a side salad **Why?** By removing the batter you reduce the amount of harmful fats and carbs	**Best:** Broiled fish with salad **Why?** Broiling is a much healthier cooking method than pan-frying. This is one of the healthiest meals there is and excellent for getting rid of cellulite
Bad: Deep-fried sweet and sour Chinese take-out **Why?** The poorest quality protein you can get, plus coated in sugar and full of bad trans fats	**Better:** Beef stir-fry with boiled rice **Why?** A good combination of vegetables and protein, but choose brown rice for added health benefits	**Best:** Chicken stir-fry with green vegetables **Why?** The perfect high-nutrient, low-calorie meal

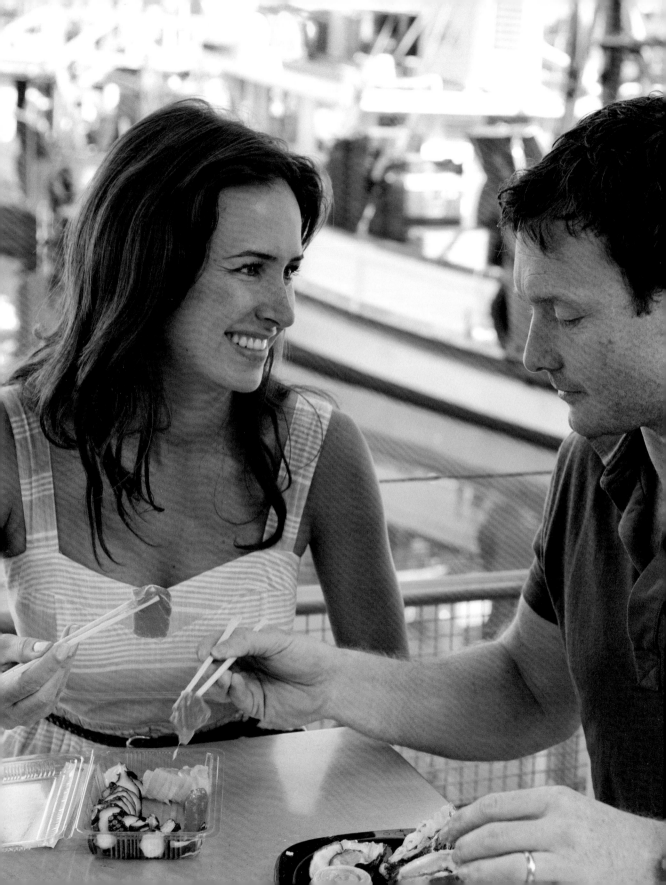

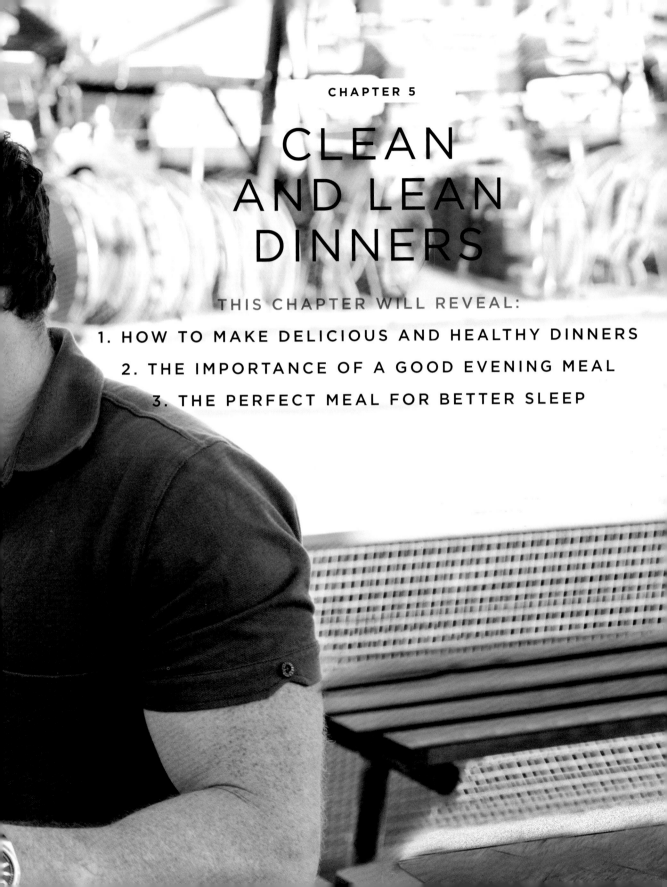

CHAPTER 5

CLEAN AND LEAN DINNERS

THIS CHAPTER WILL REVEAL:

1. HOW TO MAKE DELICIOUS AND HEALTHY DINNERS

2. THE IMPORTANCE OF A GOOD EVENING MEAL

3. THE PERFECT MEAL FOR BETTER SLEEP

One of my favorite times to eat is in the evening. I have more time than at breakfast or lunch, so I can spend longer preparing and enjoying the meal. I also love to sit with Christiane and process my day. Your evening meal shouldn't be rushed or stressful—it should be a part of your wind-down toward sleep so keep it relaxed, informal, and happy.

THE IMPORTANCE OF A GOOD DINNER

Dinner can be a lot of people's downfall. You may be full of good intentions at the start of the day and have a healthy breakfast, followed by sensible snacks and a good lunch. But come dinner time, you're likely to be tired from work and in a hurry to eat something quickly before crashing in front of the TV and then going to bed.

That's why many of us eat carb-heavy, easy-to-make dinners such as pasta or take-out pizza. But spend a little time on your dinner and your body will thank you for it. You don't have to spend hours in the kitchen after a hard day at work, but just make sure you always have the following in your kitchen—some clean and lean protein (in the form of chicken, fish, shrimp, steak, etc.), lots of herbs and spices (they add flavor to your food and have plenty of health benefits), and a huge mix of vegetables. All of the meals in this chapter are a variation on these three things.

How to ensure a good night's sleep

At dinner time, try to avoid tea, coffee, and chocolate. All contain caffeine and will disrupt your sleep. Your breakfast and lunch should rev up your energy levels to get you through the day, but the evenings are a time to wind your body down and prepare it for a good night's sleep. Remember, the better you sleep, the better your metabolism will work, and the better you'll look.

THE CLEAN & LEAN EVENING RULES

Here are my dinner rules:

1 When it comes to your evening meal, include some clean and lean protein (such as fish, steak, chicken, turkey, or eggs) and some vegetables. Please don't have a carbohydrate-only dinner, like pasta or pizza, because it will leave you feeling bloated and uncomfortable and make it harder for you to fall asleep.

2 Don't eat anything too rich, heavy, or spicy too close to bedtime. It's a myth that eating late at night will make you fat (eating the wrong thing at any time of day will make you fat), but it may disrupt your sleep. There's a strong link between good sleep and weight loss... if you don't get enough sleep, hormonal changes take place that make you hungrier (especially for sugar) and your metabolism won't work as efficiently.

3 Relax before bed. The lead up to bedtime isn't a time for work, stress, excessive TV or laptop use, or any other things that cause you to become wound up and anxious. Instead, read a good book, take a bath (pour in some relaxing oil, like lavender, or some Epsom salts to help your body shed toxins), have a calming herbal tea like chamomile, and try to get an early night. Remember, sleep before midnight is more restorative than sleep after midnight.

*top tip

If dinner is always a rush, have pre-cooked protein in your fridge ready for when you get home. Serve with crudités and a drizzle of olive oil and you have a meal in minutes

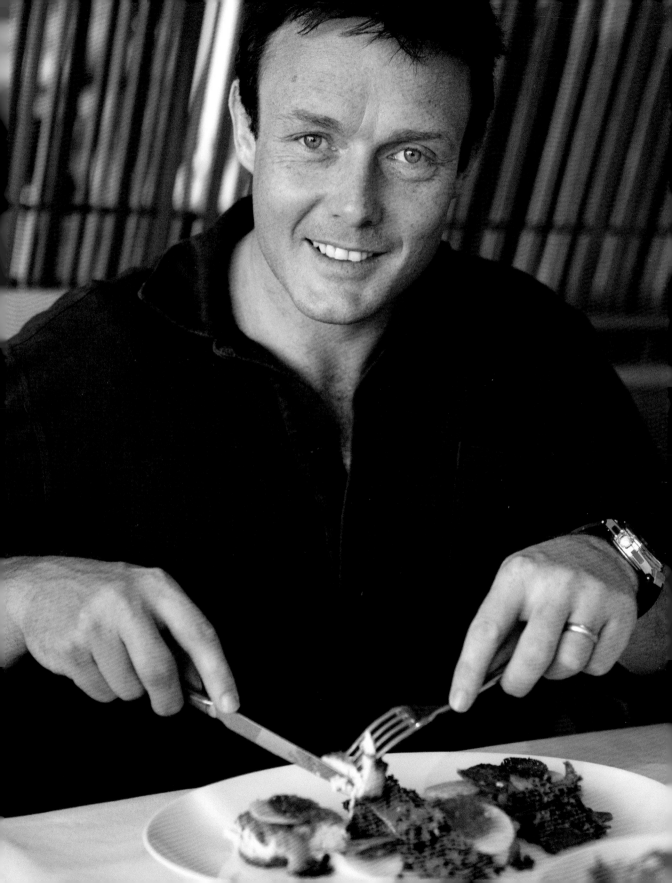

*top tip

This would go great with any broiled meat or oily fish. You can substitute goat cheese for the feta if you prefer

Roast Squash with Feta, Pumpkin Seeds, and Sprouting Broccoli

Serves 4

Ingredients

1 large acorn or butternut squash
2 tablespoons olive oil
1 teaspoon chile flakes
1 teaspoon cumin seeds
sea salt and freshly ground black pepper
2 cups purple sprouting broccoli
1½ cups pumpkin seeds, toasted
extra virgin olive oil, for drizzling
1⅓ cups feta cheese

Method

1. Preheat the oven to 400°F.

2. Peel and cut the squash into wedges or large chunks, then toss in the olive oil, chile flakes, cumin seeds, and salt and pepper.

3. Transfer to a roasting pan and roast in the preheated oven for approximately 35-45 minutes or until slightly golden and cooked.

4. Meanwhile, blanch the broccoli in salted boiling water for approximately 4 minutes, or until al dente. Once cooked, toss with the squash and pumpkin seeds.

5. Serve with a drizzle of extra virgin olive oil and the feta crumbled over the top.

Spinach and Vegetable Soup

Serves 4

Ingredients

1 carrot
4 asparagus spears
½ cup broccoli
2 large handfuls of fresh spinach
1 zucchini
2 cups organic chicken or vegetable stock
1½ tablespoons water
2 garlic cloves
¼ onion
squeeze of lemon juice
basil or other herbs, to taste
1 x 14oz can chickpeas

Method

1. Steam the carrot, asparagus, broccoli, spinach, and zucchini over a pan of boiling water for 4–5 minutes.

2. Blend all the ingredients together except the chickpeas until the desired consistency is reached, then add chickpeas for 10 seconds or keep whole.

3. Transfer to a pan and heat through until the soup is just about to simmer, and serve.

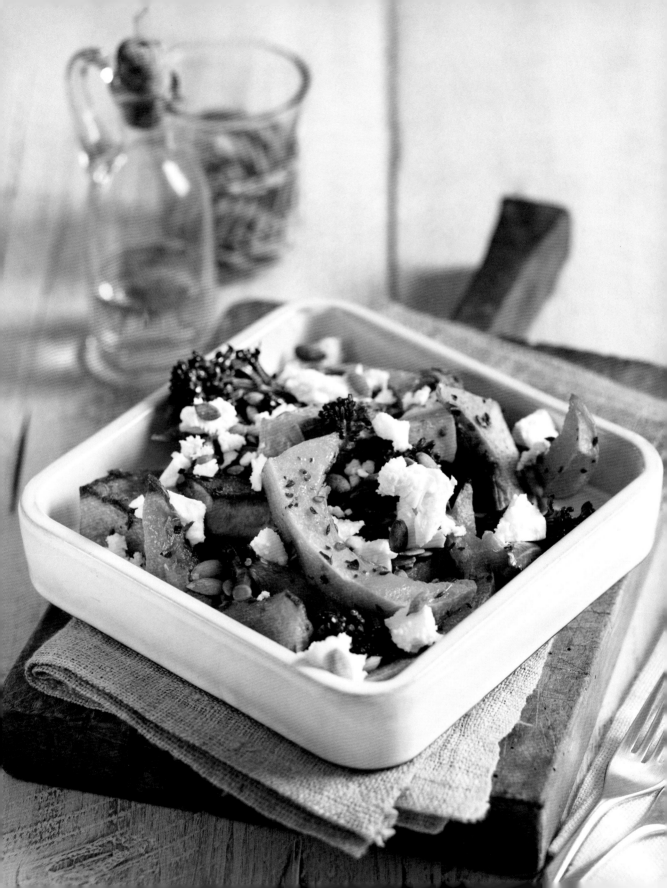

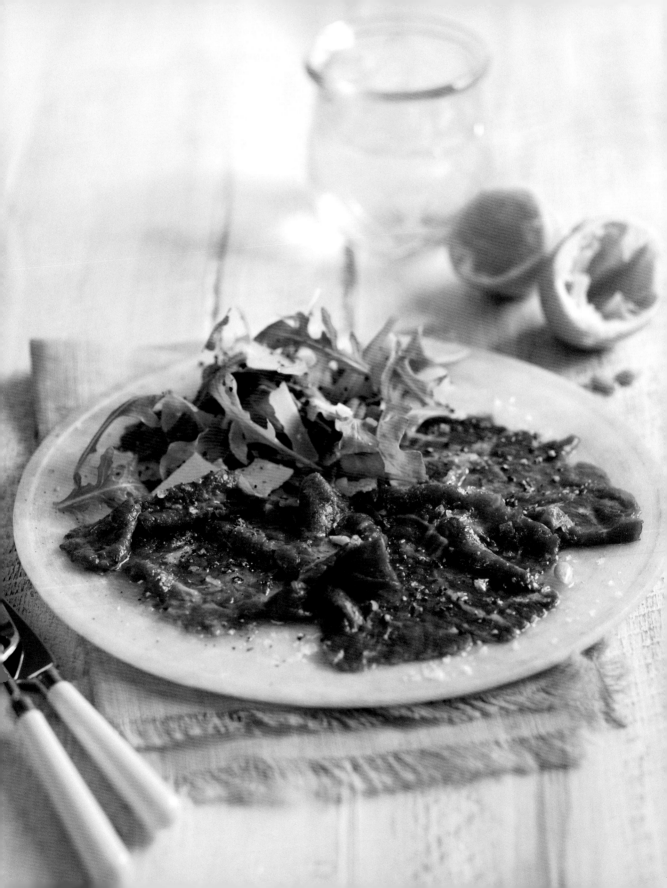

Chickpea and Carrot Stew

Serves 4

Ingredients
2 tablespoons extra virgin olive oil, plus
extra for drizzling
2 onions, chopped
2 garlic cloves, thinly sliced
1 teaspoon ground coriander
1 teaspoon ground cinnamon
1 teaspoon cumin seeds
1 teaspoon turmeric
1 teaspoon chile flakes
1 tablespoon tomato paste
1 tablespoon sherry vinegar
2 cups dried chickpeas
3 carrots, sliced
2 cups organic vegetable or chicken stock
sea salt and freshly ground black pepper
9oz baby spinach
a bunch of parsley, chopped

Method
1. Heat the oil in a large pan, add the onions and garlic, and cook gently until softened.

2. Add the spices and cook for 3 minutes.

3. Add the tomato paste and sherry vinegar and simmer for 3 minutes. Add the chickpeas and carrots, stock, and salt and pepper. Bring to steady simmer and cook for 30 minutes.

4. Finally, stir in the spinach and cook for another 3 minutes until it is wilted, then serve with the parsley and extra virgin olive oil on top.

*top tip
Chickpeas are a fantastic source
of protein and will keep you
full for hours

Angus Beef Carpaccio with Arugula Salad and Parmesan Shavings

Serves 4

Ingredients
12oz beef tenderloin
1oz piece of Parmesan
2 cups arugula
generous pinch of sea salt and freshly
ground black pepper
⅓ cup extra virgin olive oil, plus extra
for drizzling
2 lemons

Method
1. Trim and cut the beef tenderloin into about 16 slices. Tenderize the beef between plastic sheets until paper thin. Layer the thin pieces of beef on a plate in a round shape.

2. Shave the Parmesan, using a vegetable peeler to ensure nice long, thin pieces.

3. Wash and dry the arugula and season with salt and a little olive oil. Add to the carpaccio plate.

4. Squeeze the lemons into a bowl and add the extra virgin olive oil. Season and mix until smooth. Pour the dressing over the prepared carpaccio and arugula salad and top with the Parmesan shavings. Finish with sea salt and black pepper and a drizzle of extra virgin olive oil.

Broiled Chicken/ Turkey and Radicchio Salad

Serves 4

Ingredients
2 chicken or turkey breasts
2 tablespoons olive oil
sea salt and freshly ground black pepper
1 large radicchio, shredded
1 red onion, very finely sliced
a bunch of parsley, leaves separated and roughly chopped
2 tablespoons walnut oil
juice of ½ lemon
1 orange, peeled and sliced

Method
1. Preheat the broiler.

2. Place the chicken or turkey breast on a baking sheet. Rub with olive oil, salt, and pepper, then broil for roughly 10 minutes on each side, until cooked. Let cool slightly before cutting on an angle.

3. Toss the chicken with the radicchio, red onion, and parsley.

4. Dress with the walnut oil, lemon juice, salt, and pepper. Scatter the orange slices over the top and serve.

Bean Sprout Salad with Lemon Dressing

Serves 4

Ingredients
4 cups bean sprouts
1 carrot, chopped
½ yellow bell pepper, chopped
½ red/white cabbage, finely shredded

For the lemon dressing
juice of 1 lemon
4½ tablespoons olive oil
2 garlic cloves, minced
sea salt and freshly ground black pepper, to taste

Method
1. Chop all the salad ingredients and put in a bowl.

2. Mix all the dressing ingredients together then drizzle over the salad and season to taste.

*top tip
Lemons are a very "clean" fruit and help your body to eliminate toxins, so squirt some fresh lemon juice over your meals

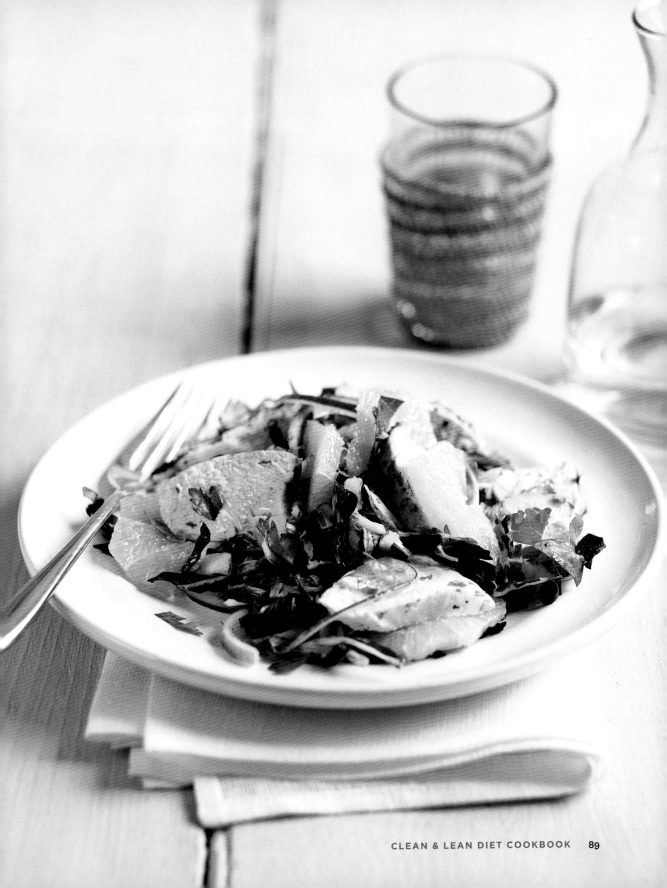

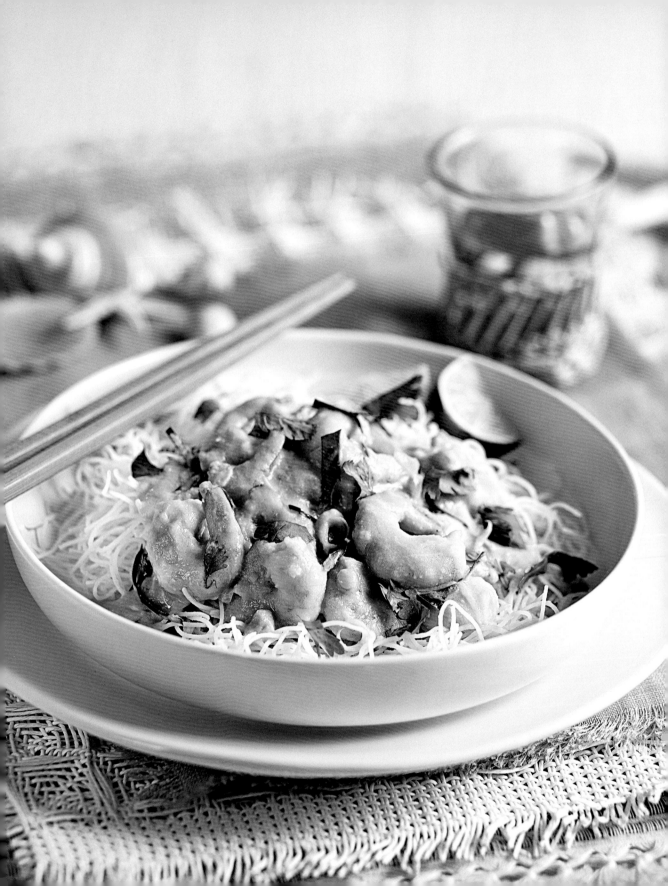

Lemongrass and Coconut Shrimp with Glass Noodles

Serves 4

Ingredients

20 large shrimp, raw and unpeeled
2 tablespoons sesame oil
2 garlic cloves, crushed
2 lemongrass stalks, very finely chopped
2in piece of fresh ginger, peeled and grated
1 green chile, finely sliced
1¾oz creamed coconut
2 kaffir lime leaves, shredded
2 tablespoons tamari soy sauce
1 tablespoon fish sauce
9oz glass rice noodles
a bunch of cilantro, to garnish
1 lime, quartered, to garnish

Method

1. Rinse the shrimp under cold water.

2. In a wok, heat the oil and gently cook the garlic, lemongrass, ginger, and chile until well softened. Add the creamed coconut, ½ cup boiling water, and the kaffir lime leaves. The sauce should be of a thick consistency. Simmer for approximately 5 minutes; do not allow to boil.

3. Add the shrimp and continue to cook until they have turned pink.

4. Add the tamari and fish sauce and taste. Add more of both if needed to adjust the flavor.

5. Meanwhile, cook the noodles according to the package instructions.

6. Serve the shrimp over the noodles, sprinkled with cilantro and a wedge of lime on the side.

*top tip

Ginger is good for your digestive health and can help your body break down fatty foods

Try to eat fish at least two or three times a week. Studies show that it lowers your risk of heart disease, boosts your IQ and concentration, and it's a fantastic source of healthy protein that keeps hunger at bay. Oily fish, such as salmon and mackerel, contain more fat and calories than white fish like cod, but they also contain more omega-3 fatty acids. These essential fats actually help your body burn fat more efficiently, plus they boost brain power. Try to vary the fish you eat each week— visit your fishmonger (most supermarkets have them) and ask them what fresh fish they have in that week. They'll also give you tips on how to cook it and the vegetables it goes best with

Whole Baked Sea Bass
Serves 4

Ingredients
2 whole sea bass, approximately 1lb 2oz each (I think the smaller tastes fresher)
4 tablespoons olive oil, plus extra for drizzling
1 lemon
½ thumb-sized piece of fresh ginger
sea salt and freshly ground black pepper
steamed spinach and green beans, to serve

Method
1. Preheat the oven to 350°F.

2. Clean the sea bass and rub in the oil, both inside and out. Wash and chop the lemon and ginger, then put inside the fish. Add salt and pepper.

3. Place the sea bass in an ovenproof dish and cover with foil, then bake in the preheated oven for 20-25 minutes. When ready, the skin and bones should fall off easily.

4. Serve with the greens and drizzle some olive oil over the top.

*top tip
Don't be scared to cook a whole fish. It's one of the easiest meals you can make. Just stuff it with clean and lean flavors, like herbs and lemon, and bake it in foil. Simple!

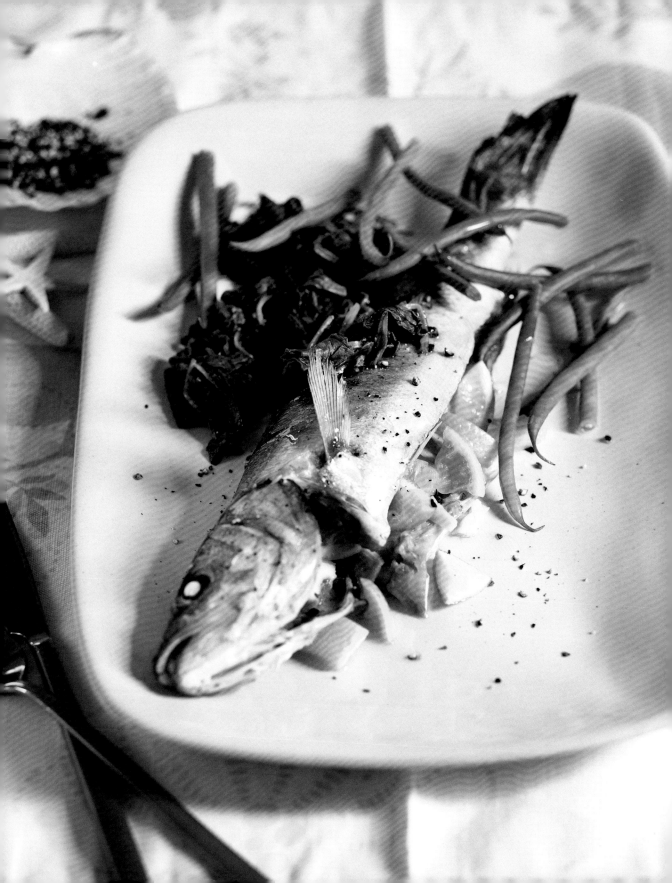

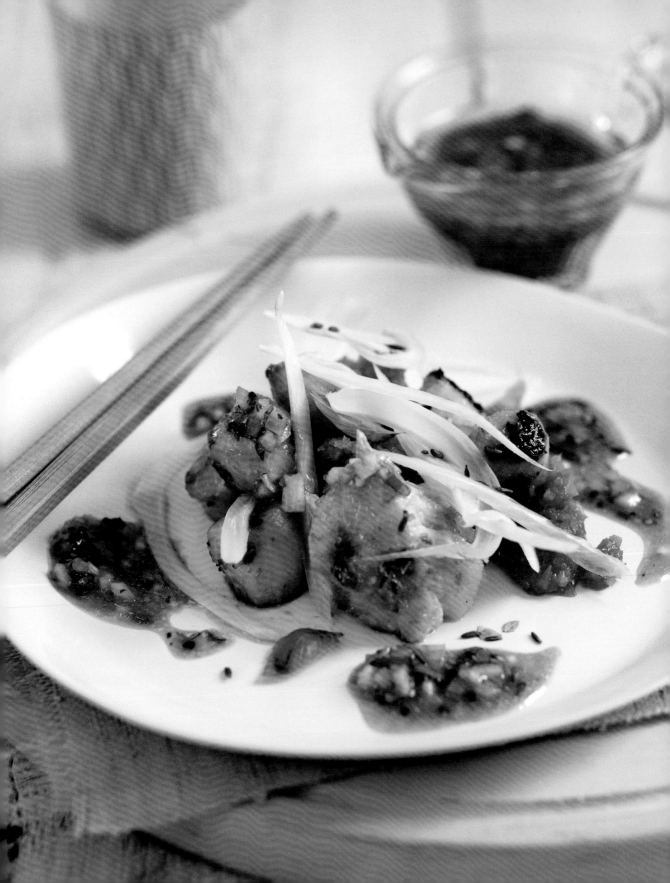

White Miso Scallops

Serves 4

Ingredients
2 carrots, sliced
¾ cup organic carrot juice
4 baby fennel, sliced paper thin
2 teaspoons white miso paste
20 small sea scallops
olive oil
2 tablespoons good-quality white
wine vinegar, to season
1 teaspoon cumin seeds, lightly toasted
a handful of small basil leaves, to garnish

For the dressing
1 teaspoon whole-grain mustard
juice of 2 lemons
½ cup fresh tomato juice
1 small Spanish onion, finely chopped
2 tablespoons extra virgin olive oil
sea salt and freshly ground black pepper
1 tablespoon snipped basil or tarragon leaves

Method

1. Place the carrots in a medium-sized saucepan along with the carrot juice. Bring to a boil, then reduce the heat to a nice, steady simmer.

2. While the carrots are cooking, prepare the dressing. Whisk together the mustard and lemon juice in a bowl, then stir in all the other ingredients, except for the herbs.

3. Place the fennel in a bowl of iced water. This will firm it up nicely.

4. When the carrots are cooked, place them in a blender along with their juice and process to a smooth consistency. Pass through a fine sieve and adjust the seasoning to your liking.

5. Rub the miso paste over the scallops and let rest for 5 minutes.

6. Heat the carrot purée in a pan over low heat.

7. Heat a non-stick frying pan to high heat. Add a little olive oil and give it a swirl. Add the scallops to the pan and let them caramelize. Flip the scallops over and leave them to caramelize on the second side.

8. Remove the fennel from the iced water and place in a bowl. Season with a little of the white wine vinegar and sprinkle with the toasted cumin seeds.

9. Before serving, add the herbs to the dressing. Then put the warmed purée on a plate. Remove the scallops from the pan and place them on the purée. Serve with the fennel slices, drizzled with a little dressing and garnished with the basil leaves.

*top tip

Scallops are a rich source of omega 3, which can also help ease symptoms of premenstrual syndrome

Seared Sirloin with Arugula and Watercress Salad

Serves 4

Ingredients
2 sirloin steaks
2 tablespoons olive oil
sea salt and freshly ground black pepper
a bunch of arugula
a bunch of watercress
10 cherry tomatoes, halved

For the dressing
a small bunch of tarragon, finely chopped
a small bunch of basil, finely chopped
4 tablespoons extra virgin olive oil
juice of 1 lemon
1 tablespoon white wine vinegar
sea salt and freshly ground black pepper
3½oz piece Parmigiano-Reggiano

Method
1. Heat a grill pan until very hot.

2. Rub the steaks with the olive oil and salt and pepper, and sear in the heated pan for 2–3 minutes on each side for medium-rare. Let rest for 5–10 minutes.

3. Meanwhile, to make the dressing, whisk together the herbs, extra virgin olive oil, lemon juice, vinegar, salt, and pepper.

4. Toss the greens and tomatoes in the dressing. Slice the steaks very thinly on an angle and lay over the salad. Finally, shave the Parmigiano-Reggiano over the top.

Seared Wasabi and Sesame Tuna with Chile and Green Beans

Serves 4

Ingredients
1 tablespoon wasabi paste
1 tablespoon sesame seeds
1 teaspoon olive oil
4 tuna steaks
1 tablespoon sesame oil
2 red chiles, finely sliced
1 teaspoon black onion seeds
2 cups green beans, trimmed and blanched
1 tablespoon oyster sauce
1 lime, cut into wedges, to serve

Method
1. Heat a grill pan until very hot.

2. Mix together the wasabi paste, sesame seeds, and olive oil and rub over the tuna steaks. Sear the tuna for 2–3 minutes on each side, then let cool.

3. In a frying pan, heat the sesame oil, add the chiles and onion seeds, toss for 2–3 minutes, then add the beans and the oyster sauce. Continue to cook for another 5–8 minutes, then serve with the tuna and lime wedges.

*top tip

Red meat is an excellent source of iron— great for boosting energy levels— but only have it once or twice a week because it contains saturated fat

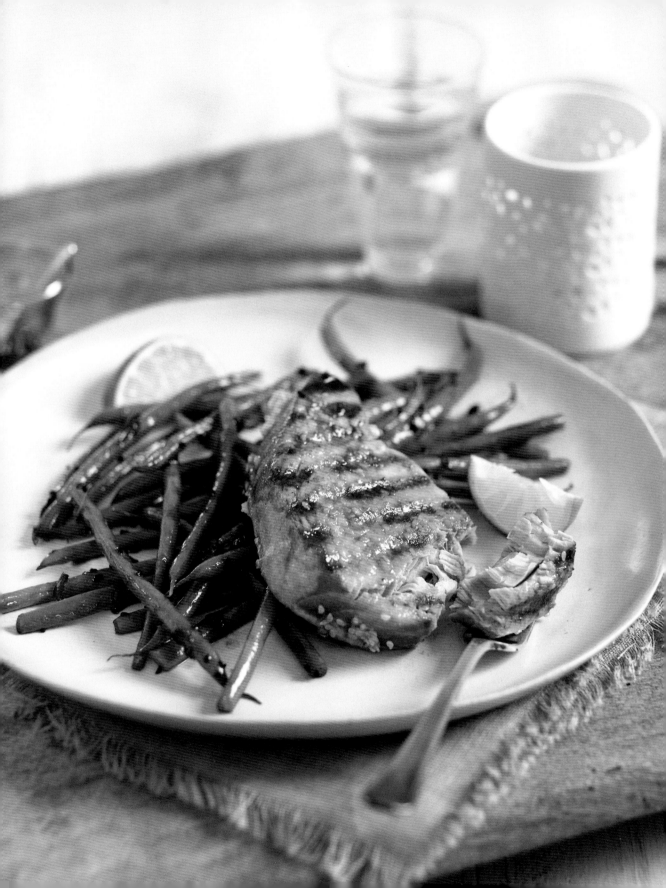

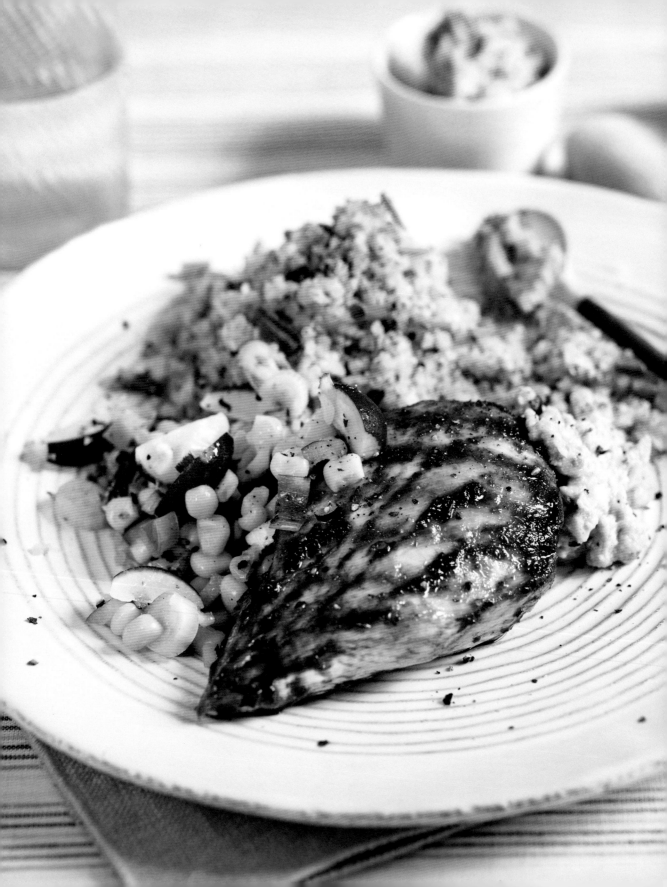

Grilled Cajun Chicken

Serves 4

Ingredients

4 x 4½oz boneless, skinless chicken breasts
sea salt and freshly ground black pepper
2 tablespoons harissa paste
1 cup quinoa
1 tablespoon olive oil
1 cup boiling water
a few chives, chopped
1 ripe avocado, peeled and pitted
juice of ½ lemon, or to taste

For the salsa

1 cob sweet corn, kernels cut off the cob
2 red radishes, cut into quarters
⅔ cup red onion, finely chopped
1 scallion, sliced
olive oil
juice of 1 lime

Method

1. Preheat the oven to 350°F.

2. Season the chicken breasts with salt and pepper, then grill so that there are nice grill marks on the breasts. Rub the harissa paste over the surface of the chicken and place in the oven until cooked; this will take about 6–8 minutes. Set aside to rest.

3. Toast the quinoa in a hot pan until it takes on a slight golden brown color, then remove from the heat immediately, place in a mixing bowl, add the olive oil and boiling water just to cover, place plastic wrap over the top, and allow to steam. Once cooled, add the chopped chives to the cooked quinoa.

4. For the salsa, combine the corn kernels, radish, red onion, sliced scallion, olive oil, and lime juice. Season to taste.

5. Place the ripe avocado in a food-processor and pulse until smooth, adding seasoning and lemon juice to taste.

*top tip

Salmon is a good source of healthy fat, which can help your body burn fat—especially around your waist. Have it at least once a week

Grilled Salmon and Green Beans with Coconut and Black Mustard seeds

Serves 4

Ingredients

4 skinless salmon fillets
sea salt and freshly ground black pepper
2 cups trimmed green beans
1 teaspoon coconut oil
2 tablespoons black mustard seeds
2 tablespoons unsweetened coconut

Method

1. Preheat the broiler.

2. Season the salmon fillets with salt and pepper, then place on a baking sheet and broil for roughly 10 minutes.

3. Blanch the beans in boiling salted water for 5–6 minutes, until al dente.

4. In a deep frying pan, heat the oil and cook the mustard seeds and coconut. After several minutes, add the beans and toss until well coated. Serve with the salmon.

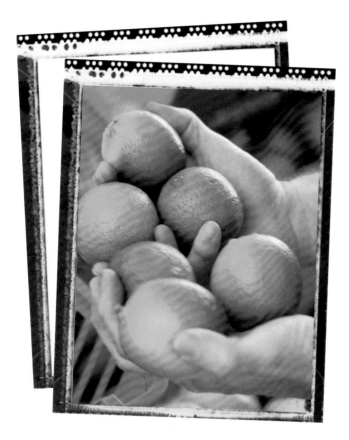

Poached Chicken/ Turkey with Herbed Brown Rice
Serves 4

Ingredients
4 chicken or small turkey breasts
1 quart organic vegetable stock
1 bay leaf
1 small onion
1 carrot
1 celery rib
1½ cups brown rice
a small bunch of parsley
a small bunch of tarragon
a small bunch of dill
3 tablespoons flaxseed oil
juice of 1 lime
sea salt and freshly ground black pepper
9oz spinach

Method
1. Place the chicken or turkey breasts in a pan with the vegetable stock, the bay leaf, onion, carrot, and celery. Bring to a gentle simmer until cooked, approximately 15 minutes.

2. Cook the rice according to package instructions, then mix with the herbs, oil, lime juice, salt, and pepper.

3. Steam the spinach over a pan of boiling water and serve the chicken on top of it with the rice.

*top tip

Poaching doesn't require any oil or fat and the result is a succulent, tender chicken

Poached Baby Chicken

Serves 4

Ingredients

1 baby chicken (approximately 14oz), giblets removed

2½ quarts organic chicken stock

1 bulb fresh garlic, cut through the center

1 carrot, cut into 2in pieces

1 leek, cut into 1¼in pieces

6 fresh parsley sprigs

1 bay leaf

3 whole white peppercorns

6 sprigs of fresh thyme

1 cup brussels sprouts, peeled and halved

½ cup organic pearl barley, rinsed

½ cup organic buckwheat, rinsed

2 tablespoons extra virgin olive oil, for frying

8 medium-sized shiitake mushrooms, stalks removed

2 celery ribs, cut into 2in stalks

⅓ cup frozen peas, defrosted

Method

1. Place the chicken in a pan and cover with the stock.

2. Add the garlic, carrot, leek, parsley sprigs, bay leaf, peppercorns, and thyme. Bring up the heat, but do not boil. Let the chicken simmer very gently for 20 minutes. Once cooked, remove the chicken from the liquid and refrigerate, reserving the stock.

3. Strain the stock through a fine sieve and return to a clean pan. Bring the stock up to a simmer. Add the brussels sprouts and boil for 4–5 minutes, then remove and refresh using cold water.

4. Add the barley and buckwheat to the stock and continue cooking.

5. Remove the chicken from the fridge, ensuring it is completely chilled. Remove the breasts leaving the bone on. Trim the bone and do the same with the legs.

6. When the barley and buckwheat are cooked, strain and reserve the stock.

7. Bring the stock to a boil and reduce down to ¾ cup. Season lightly, as this will be used as a sauce to garnish your dish with and to cook the celery and peas.

8. Season the chicken breasts and legs and fry off in a little extra virgin olive oil, along with the brussels sprouts. At the same time, broil the shiitake mushrooms.

9. Heat the barley and buckwheat mixture and season to taste. Heat the reserved stock and lightly poach the celery in it. When almost cooked, add the peas.

10. Place the barley and buckwheat in the center of a serving plate, arrange the chicken pieces on top, and garnish with the mushrooms, peas, celery, and brussels sprouts. Serve immediately.

*top tip
Always ensure your chicken is piping hot and white (with no pink bits) throughout

Oven-poached Salmon

Serves 4

Ingredients
4 large organic salmon fillets, skinned and boned
a large bunch of dill
4 lemons, each sliced into 6
sea salt and freshly ground black pepper
extra virgin olive oil, for drizzling
asparagus, green beans, or spinach, for serving

Method
1. Preheat the oven to 350°F.

2. On a large sheet of parchment paper, (tin foil will also work), place the salmon and lay the dill sprigs, lemon slices, salt, and pepper and drizzle with olive oil. If you have any white wine open, a splash is a delicious addition.

3. Fold the paper over to make a parcel and place on a baking sheet.

4. Bake in the oven for approximately 15–20 minutes, until the fish is completely pink and flakes away.

5. Serve with steamed vegetables such as asparagus, green beans, or spinach.

Lamb Steak with Mashed Peas

Serves 4

Ingredients
4 lamb steaks
2 teaspoons olive oil
6 sprigs of thyme, chopped
pinch of sea salt and freshly ground black pepper

For the peas
2¾ cups peas
3½ tablespoons butter
4 sprigs of mint
pinch of sea salt

Method
1. Marinate the lamb steaks with the olive oil, thyme, and salt and pepper for a minimum of an hour, or overnight. Then broil them under a preheated broiler for 3–5 minutes on each side.

2. Boil the peas in water until tender, then strain and place in a blender with the butter, mint, and sea salt until it has reached a soft consistency to your liking. Serve with the broiled lamb steaks.

*top tip
Lamb contains less fat than other red meats and provides many essential nutrients

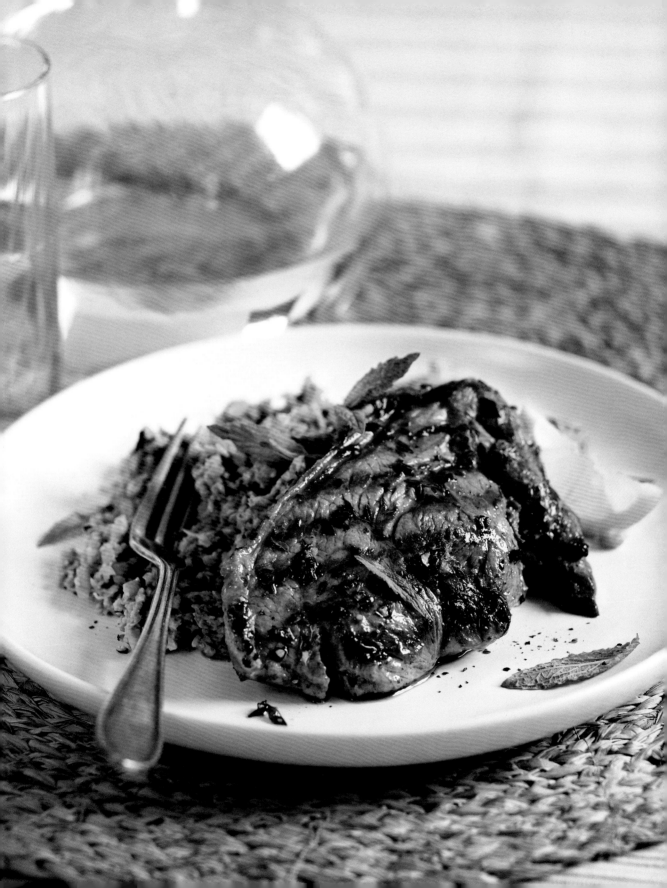

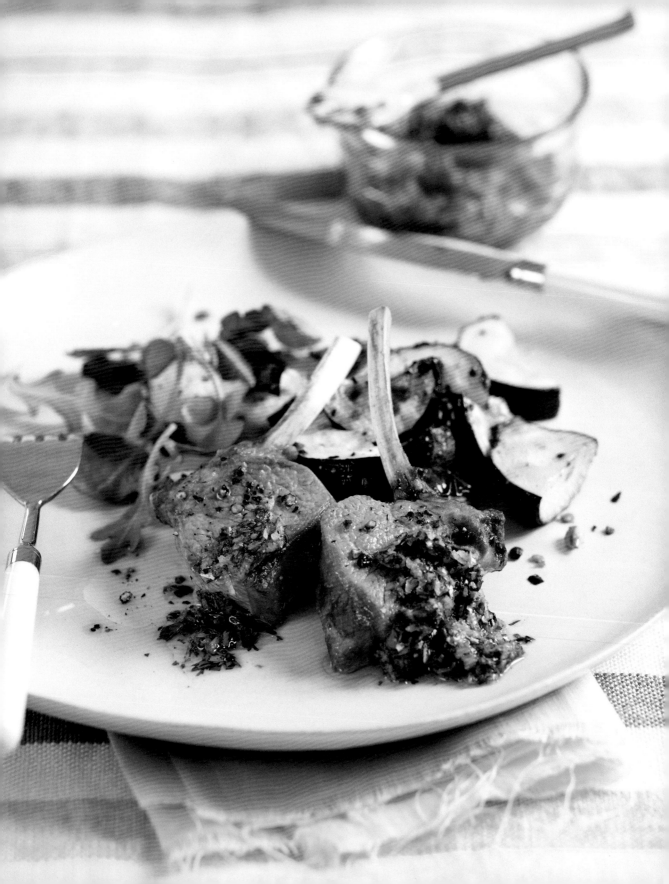

Lamb Cutlets with Chermoula Dip and Roast Zucchini

Serves 4

Ingredients

4 large zucchini

juice of 1 lemon

1 teaspoon chile flakes

sea salt and freshly ground black pepper

2 tablespoons olive oil

2 garlic cloves, peeled and crushed

8 lamb cutlets

a bunch of arugula

a bunch of watercress

For the chermoula

a bunch of parsley

a bunch of cilantro

a bunch of mint

zest of 1 lemon

3 anchovy fillets, in olive oil

2 tablespoons olive oil

sea salt and freshly ground black pepper

*top tip

You can substitute the zucchini for your favorite greens—such as beans or broccoli

Method

1. Preheat the oven to 375°F.

2. Slice the zucchini in half, lengthwise. Make a paste with the lemon juice, chile flakes, garlic, salt and pepper, and 1 tablespoon of the olive oil. Rub the paste over the zucchini, then roast them in the preheated oven for approximately 30 minutes or until cooked.

3. To make the chermoula, blend together the herbs, lemon zest, anchovies, olive oil, and salt and pepper. Adjust the seasoning if needed.

4. Preheat the broiler.

5. Rub the lamb cutlets with the remaining olive oil and salt and pepper and broil for approximately 3-4 minutes according to your taste.

6. Top the lamb with the chermoula and serve with the zucchini and with the arugula and watercress, lightly dressed with olive oil and the remaining lemon juice.

Turkey Burgers
Serves 4

Ingredients
14oz ground turkey
juice of 2 limes
4 lemongrass stalks, chopped
sea salt and freshly ground black pepper,
to taste
scallions, finely chopped
iceberg lettuce, to serve

Method

1. Preheat the broiler.

2. Simply put all the ingredients except the iceberg lettuce into a bowl and mix together. Cover and put in the fridge to marinate/ infuse for 30 minutes–1 hour.

3. Remove the burger mixture from the fridge and shape into patties. You can make these as big or as small as you like. Then place them under the broiler for 6–8 minutes on each side. (Time varies depending on the size of the burgers.)

4. Tear off the whole lettuce leaves, wash them, and then place on a plate in the middle of the table. Use these to wrap up your burgers.

5. Serve with oven-roasted vegetables.

Rosie's Lemon-roasted Chicken
Serves 4

Ingredients
1 medium chicken
1 lemon, cut in half and zested
3 garlic cloves
sea salt and freshly ground black pepper,
to taste
2 tablespoons olive oil
1 cup brown rice
1¼ cups organic chicken or vegetable stock
4½ cups kale, shredded
1 avocado, sliced

Method

1. Preheat the oven to 375°F.

2. Stuff the chicken with the lemon and garlic cloves and season with salt and pepper. Drizzle the skin with the olive oil and season well all over.

3. Roast the chicken for approximately 1½ hours.

4. Boil the brown rice in chicken or vegetable stock and steam the kale over a pan of boiling water.

5. Serve the chicken on a plate with the kale and rice and a scattering of avocado and lemon zest.

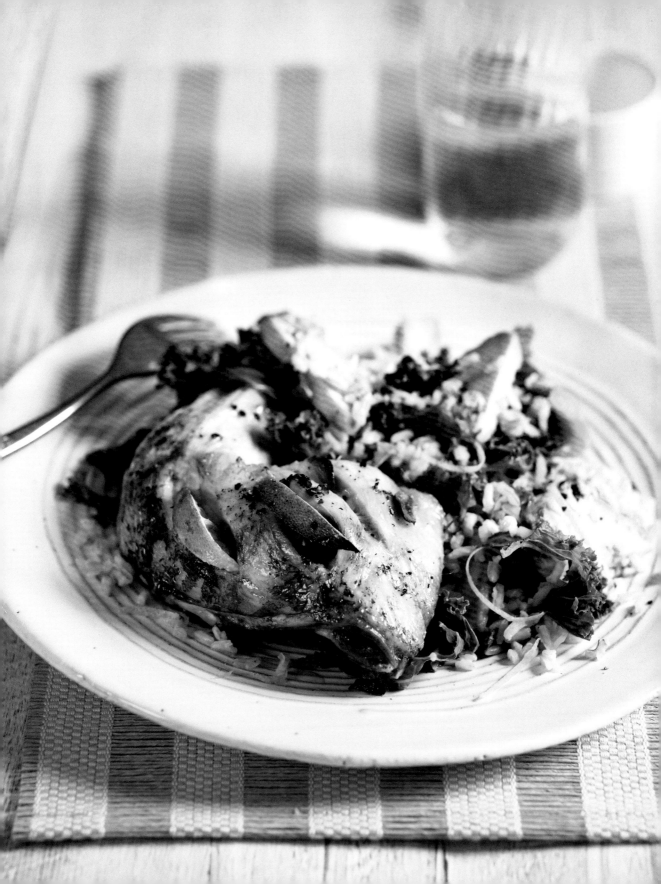

HERE'S MY HANDY "BAD, BETTER & BEST"

BAD	BETTER	BEST
Bad: Sweet honey granola **Why?** Even though honey isn't a processed sugar, it's still high GI, leading to quick-release glucose that won't keep you feeling full for long	**Better:** Oat muesli with cinnamon **Why?** Cinnamon is great at helping to regulate blood sugar levels and the muesli provides fiber to keep you feeling full	**Best:** Gluten-free oatmeal with mixed nuts and organic berries **Why?** A great blend of low GI carbohydrates, protein, and healthy fats that also contains plenty of fiber and antioxidants
Bad: Croissant with butter **Why?** Highly processed and with very little protein content	**Better:** Whole-grain bagel with hazelnut butter **Why?** Hazelnut butter is a great source of vitamin E, which helps protect the skin against aging	**Best:** Sourdough toast with sliced avocado and organic tomatoes **Why?** Avocado's high antioxidant content has been shown to benefit our health and it's yummy!
Bad: Cereal with milk, orange juice, and flavored yogurt **Why?** Highly processed and high in sodium. Full of empty calories	**Better:** Whole-grain bread with organic cashew butter **Why?** A combination of healthy fats, protein, and fiber helps keep you feel full for longer	**Best:** Spelt bread with almond butter **Why?** This is an incredibly yummy, quick snack and almond butter is a great source of essential fatty acids and protein
Bad: Sticky white rice sushi **Why?** Can irritate your digestive system, causing your tummy to bloat	**Better:** Wild rice sushi **Why?** Wild rice is naturally high in folic acid, which is a beneficial vitamin during pregnancy	**Best:** Brown rice sushi with a seaweed salad **Why?** Brown rice is a great source of magnesium, which helps you sleep better
Bad: Fat-free fruit-flavored yogurt **Why?** Full of artificial flavors and high in sugar	**Better:** Organic greek yogurt **Why?** Introduces live cultures to your digestive system, which helps maintain a flat tummy	**Best:** Organic yogurt with live cultures, organic cinnamon, and a handful of pistachios **Why?** Pistachios are a good low GI protein snack and cinnamon can help regulate blood sugar levels
Bad: Vegetable curry made with white rice and sweet sauce **Why?** White rice combined with sweet sauce can cause your blood sugar levels to rise, which makes you crave more sugar	**Better:** Vegetable curry with brown rice and cumin **Why?** Cumin can help relieve digestive disorders and is a good source of iron	**Best:** Vegetable curry made with quinoa and greek yogurt **Why?** Quinoa is an excellent source of protein for vegetarians as well as a great gluten-free choice

VEGETARIAN GUIDE:

BAD	BETTER	BEST
Bad: Canned vegetable soup with tofu and croutons **Why?** Low protein content with highly processed ingredients and high salt content	**Better:** Homemade soup with chilled fennel and halloumi **Why?** Fennel is a natural libido booster and it's delicious	**Best:** Organic homemade vegetable soup with organic chickpeas and lentils **Why?** A clean, nutritious high-protein meal and a good source of fiber
Bad: Baked cheese and tomato pasta made with canned tomatoes **Why?** A combination of high GI carbohydrate with unhealthy fats and minimal protein content	**Better:** Whole-grain pasta with fresh tomatoes **Why?** Tomatoes contain lycopene, which is an incredible antioxidant that helps fight cancerous cell formation	**Best:** Organic tomatoes and basil with rice noodles and olive oil **Why?** Basil is a great immune system booster and rice noodles don't contain gluten
Bad: Take-out vegetarian pizza **Why?** Highly processed ingredients that are high in sugar and salt	**Better:** Homemade whole wheat pizza with fresh vegetables **Why?** Fresh ingredients contain a higher nutrient and mineral content	**Best:** Gluten-free pizza with organic tomato, goat cheese, and mixed herbs **Why?** Mixed herbs have a host of antioxidants and health benefits
Bad: Peanut butter soy smoothie **Why?** Full of hydrogenated fat, which can affect your biochemistry	**Better:** Homemade smoothie made with orange juice and fruit **Why?** Much more nutrient dense foods that have a high fiber and antioxidant content	**Best:** Homemade smoothie made with rice milk, organic fruit, and nuts **Why?** Rice milk is a great lactose-free alternative to cow's milk and is easy to digest and the nuts provide protein
Bad: Soy burger with bread roll and fries **Why?** High trans-fat content and full of pesticides that can be toxic	**Better:** Quorn burger in a whole-grain roll with a garden salad **Why?** A much better source of protein with a high amount of dietary fiber to help aid digestion	**Best:** Tempeh burger (no roll) with organic roasted vegetables **Why?** A great source of protein that is incredibly nutrient dense for vegetarians
Bad: Supermarket frozen cheese quiche **Why?** Highly processed and high GI—a recipe for weight gain	**Better:** Homemade shallot tart with goat cheese **Why?** A lighter option with no artificial flavors and preservatives	**Best:** Bell peppers stuffed with mushrooms and feta cheese **Why?** Mushrooms are a good source of vitamin D

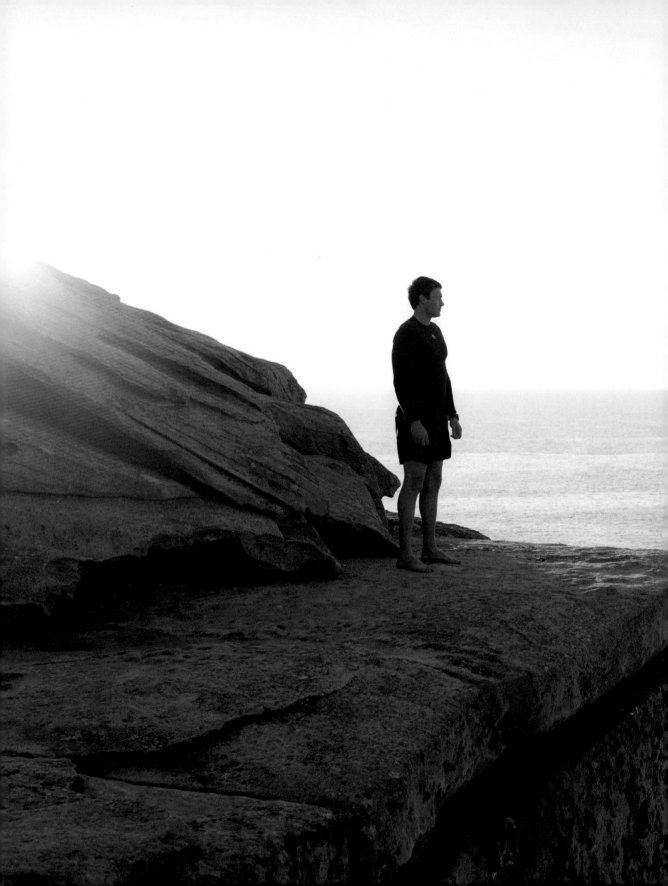

CHAPTER 6

CLEAN AND LEAN AROUND THE WORLD

THIS CHAPTER WILL REVEAL:

1. HOW OTHER COUNTRIES AND CULTURES STAY HEALTHY

2. DELICIOUS CLEAN & LEAN DISHES FROM AROUND THE WORLD

3. HOW TO COOK CLEAN & LEAN

At the very beginning of the book, I wrote about the fact that I'm Australian and how this has influenced the foods I eat and the way I cook. In Australia, eating is a very sociable experience—we love getting lots of friends together and enjoying BBQs, fresh fish, and seasonal vegetables. I'm lucky in that my work has taken me around the world and, along the way, I've learned about how other countries cook and eat. In this chapter, I'll be sharing with you some fantastic recipes I've picked up on my travels ...

Australia

The Australians love a BBQ, which is a very healthy way of cooking lovely, lean steaks and fresh fish because it allows any excess fat to drain away from the food before it reaches your tummy. They also love grilling and lightly stir-frying or steaming colorful vegetables.

The extensive Australian coastline means seafood—in particular crab, lobster, shrimp, tuna, salmon, and abalone—is readily available. They're all high in protein, with the more oily fishes packed with fat-burning and tummy-flattening essential fatty acid omega-3, which is also heart-healthy. Australian dishes often use locally grown vegetables rich in the antioxidant vitamins A and C. They typically eat seasonally, so artichokes and asparagus in spring and bell peppers and zucchini in the summer.

Thailand

While Thai food has long been ranked as one of the healthiest, the Westernized version is covered in thick, gloopy, and highly processed sauces. Thai food is traditionally prepared in a stir-fry style, and this speedy cooking approach means the food keeps a lot of its natural flavor and nutrients. They also steam a lot of their food, which also retains nutrients.

Thai dishes typically contain lots of fresh lean meat, fish, and vegetables and rely on fresh nutrient-rich herbs and spices such as turmeric, cilantro, and lemongrass. These ingredients are packed full of antioxidants and help to increase energy levels, as well as promote overall health.

The Caribbean

The hot, tropical climate of the Caribbean is great for growing fresh fruit, vegetables, and herbs. Caribbean dishes often contain fresh local fish, such as red snapper, mahi mahi, and blue marlin. Broiling, barbecuing, and steaming are popular and all are low-fat ways of cooking. In the Caribbean, fish and meats often undergo a long preparatory process in order to enhance their taste. Lean chicken, for example, is usually washed several times with water and vinegar and left overnight to marinate in a mix of fresh herbs. Natural ingredients mean that food is flavorful without artificial flavorings and colorings. Nutmeg, cinnamon, and ginger are typical flavorings found in the Caribbean.

France

French women don't stay so slim on cheese and croissants alone. In fact, the French like to keep cooking simple and use lots of fresh ingredients bought from the local markets. These natural ingredients avoid the need to use lots of artificial flavorings and additives.

While specialities differ between regions, French cuisine is centered around fresh vegetables and lots of protein. In particular, zucchini, which is low in calories and packed with vitamin C, and tomatoes, which are high in vitamins C and E, are a staple part of French dishes. Mussels, which are low in salt, fat, and cholesterol, and fresh fish are all high in protein and omega-3 fatty acids. Heart-healthy olives and olive oil are also popular.

Greece

The Greeks use lots of olive oil too, which is high in antioxidants. Dishes are often prepared "mezze-style," a Greek version of the Spanish tapas, consisting of several small dishes including vine leaves, tzatziki, Kalamata olives, and broiled meats.

The Greek diet is built around oils, nuts, grains, cheese, and vegetables, plus they take advantage of the locally grown wild greens and herbs like oregano, parsley, thyme, and basil, which are typically low in calories, full of vitamin C, and rich in folic acid. Greeks have fantastic access to fresh produce, and eat a large amount of fruit and vegetables. Fresh local fish, such as halibut, red mullet, swordfish, and octopus, which are high in protein and low in fat, are also an important part of the Greek diet.

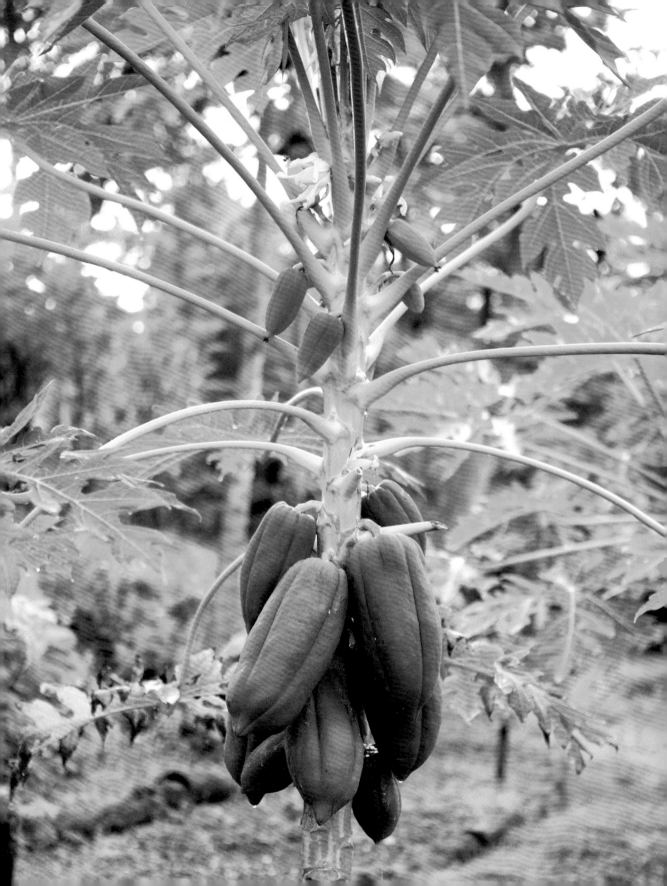

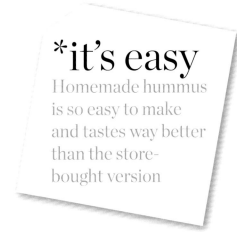

*it's easy
Homemade hummus is so easy to make and tastes way better than the store-bought version

Italian Baked Eggplant

Serves 4

Ingredients
2 large eggplants, halved
olive oil, for drizzling
sea salt and freshly ground black pepper
2 tablespoons olive oil
1 onion, finely chopped
2 garlic cloves, crushed
1 tablespoon tomato paste
1 tablespoon red wine vinegar
1 x 14oz can chopped tomatoes
2 tablespoons green olives, halved
1 tablespoon capers, rinsed
¾ cup ricotta, whisked

To serve
a bunch of arugula
a small bunch of basil

Method

1. Preheat the oven to 400°F.

2. Place the eggplant halves in an ovenproof dish and drizzle with olive oil, salt, and pepper. Place in the preheated oven and roast for approximately 35-45 minutes, or until soft.

3. Meanwhile in a pan, heat the 2 tablespoons of olive oil and gently cook the onion and garlic until soft. Increase the heat and add the tomato paste and cook for another 3-4 minutes. Add the vinegar and simmer for 2 minutes. Now add the chopped tomatoes and some salt and pepper. Bring to a steady simmer and cook for 15-20 minutes. Add the olives and capers and adjust the seasoning, if needed.

4. Spoon the sauce over the eggplants and top with the ricotta. Return to the oven for another 10 minutes before serving on the arugula with basil leaves scattered over the top.

Hummus

Serves 4

Ingredients
1¼ cups dried chickpeas
3-5 tablespoons lemon juice, to taste
1½ tablespoons tahini
2 garlic cloves, crushed
½ teaspoon sea salt
2 tablespoons olive oil, plus more for garnish
parsley, to garnish (optional)

Method

1. Soak the chickpeas overnight in cold water, then boil until soft (approximately 1 hour), but not mashed. Drain and reserve the liquid, then let cool.

2. Combine the remaining ingredients in a blender or food processor. Add ½ cup of the reserved liquid from the chickpeas. Blend for 3-5 minutes on low until thoroughly mixed and smooth.

3. Transfer to a serving bowl and create a shallow well in the center of the hummus.

4. Pour a small amount (1-2 tablespoons) of olive oil in the well and garnish with parsley (optional). Serve immediately with fresh, warm or toasted pita bread, or cover and refrigerate.

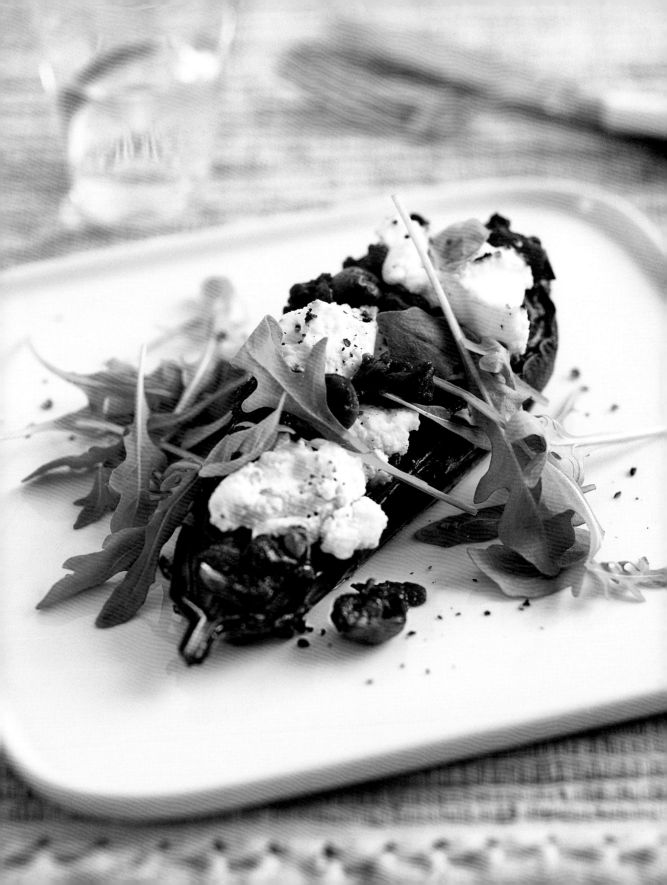

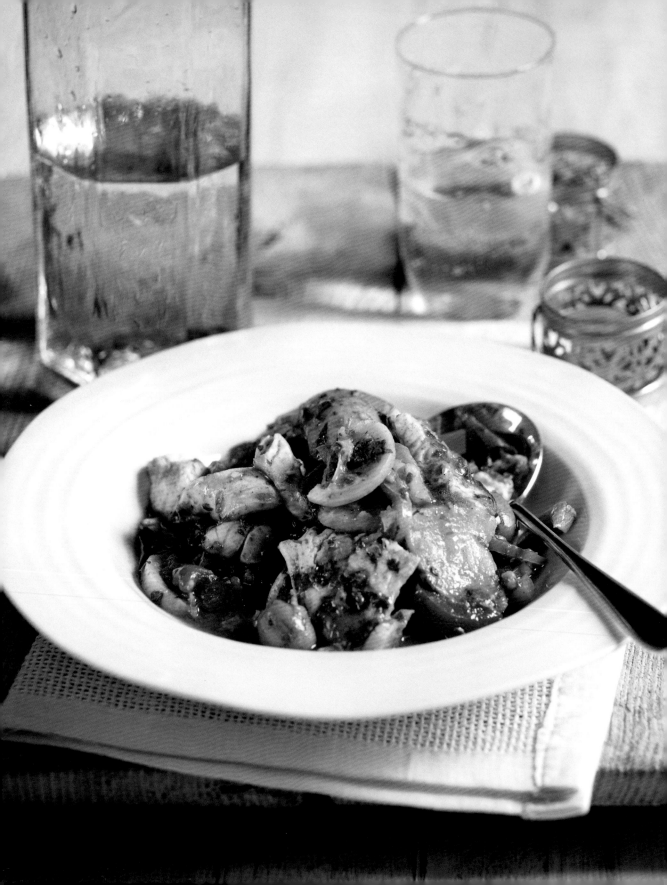

*top tip

A recent study found that cilantro can help treat the effects of food poisoning. In fact, several herbs have healing properties: Mint helps improve digestion, thyme can soothe sore throats and reduces coughs, rosemary helps boost the circulation and aids digestion, parsley, full of vitamin C and iron, can help improve immunity, and cinnamon, full of health-boosting antioxidants, can keep your blood sugar levels steady, which prevents sugar cravings

Grouper Tagine

Serves 4

Ingredients
1lb 10oz grouper fillets
2¼lb new potatoes
2 red bell peppers
2 green bell peppers
2 large tomatoes
2 lemons
2 tablespoons olive oil
green olives and pickled lemon, to garnish

For the marinade (chermoula)
1 lemon
3 garlic cloves
a bunch of parsley
a bunch of cilantro
sea salt and freshly ground black pepper
1 teaspoon paprika
1 teaspoon cumin
1 teaspoon cinnamon
¼ cup olive oil

Method

1. Cut the grouper fillets into four equal-sized slices.

2. For the chermoula, squeeze the juice from the lemon, crush the garlic cloves, chop the parsley and cilantro, and mix together. Season with salt and pepper and add the paprika, cumin, cinnamon, and olive oil. Mix and add the fish. Leave for about 1 hour.

3. Meanwhile, peel the potatoes and cut into slices.

4. Wash the red and green bell peppers and cut into strips. Wash the tomatoes and slice the lemons.

5. Heat the olive oil in a saucepan and add the potatoes. Add the marinated grouper and the remaining chermoula and pour in a glass (about 6½fl oz) of water.

6. Add the peppers and lemon slices and simmer over low heat for about 30 minutes. Add the tomatoes and continue to cook for 15 minutes. Arrange in a tagine dish and garnish with the green olives and zest of pickled lemon.

Persian Pomegranate Lamb Kofte with Buckwheat

Serves 4

Ingredients
14oz lean ground lamb
2 garlic cloves, crushed
a bunch of cilantro, leaves and roots separated and chopped
1 small red onion, finely chopped
1 green chile, seeded and sliced
2 tablespoons pomegranate syrup
sea salt and freshly ground black pepper
¾ cup buckwheat
a bunch of parsley, chopped
1 small cucumber, seeded and diced
¾ cup pine nuts, toasted
seeds of 1 pomegranate
2 tablespoons flaxseed oil
juice of 1 lemon
plain yogurt, to serve

Method

1. In a food-processor, blend the lamb, garlic, cilantro roots, red onion, chile, pomegranate syrup, and salt and pepper.

2. Once well blended, shape into small balls (should make roughly 16-20).

3. Meanwhile, soak the buckwheat in boiling water, just covering it. Let sit for 15-20 minutes, then fluff up with a fork.

4. Preheat the broiler. Place the lamb kofte on a wire rack on a baking sheet and broil for 4-5 minutes before turning and repeating.

5. Mix the buckwheat with the parsley, cilantro leaves, cucumber, pine nuts, and pomegranate seeds. Dress with the oil and lemon juice and season with salt and pepper.

6. Serve the kofte on the buckwheat salad with a spoonful of plain yogurt.

Balinese Steamed Fish

Serves 4

Ingredients
a small bunch of cilantro, roots on
zest of 1 lime
1 green chile, seeded and finely chopped
2 garlic cloves, peeled and crushed
2 kaffir lime leaves
1in piece of ginger, peeled and finely chopped
2 lemongrass stalks, tough outer leaves removed, smashed and chopped finely
1 teaspoon turmeric
1 tablespoon oil, any type
sea salt and freshly ground black pepper
either 4 whole mackerel or 8 sardines, gutted and cleaned, heads on or off or 4 fillets of white fish, such as hake, red snapper, or haddock
4 small banana leaves, or 1 split into 4, large enough to wrap around the fish
spinach or bok choy, to serve

Method

1. Preheat the oven to 350°F.

2. In a food-processor, blend all the ingredients apart from the fish and banana leaves, until you have a thick paste.

3. Lay the fish in the separate banana leaves and rub the paste over the top—a thick layer is good.

4. Wrap the banana leaves around the fish to create a snug package and tie with string. Place on a wire rack over a roasting pan filled with hot water. Bake in the preheated oven for roughly 15 minutes, then untie the parcel to check that the fish is cooked—it should be firm to touch and completely white, not translucent.

5. Serve with some spinach or bok choy.

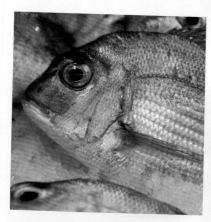
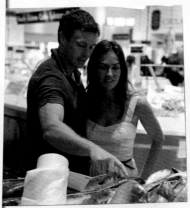
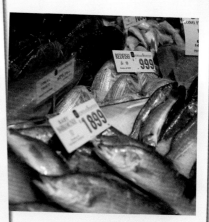
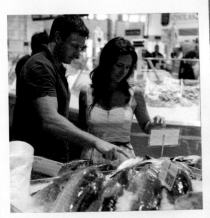
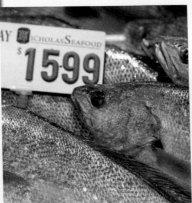
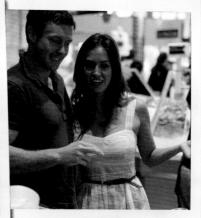
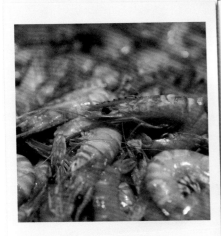
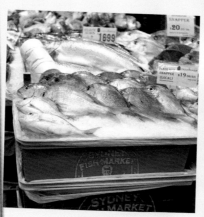
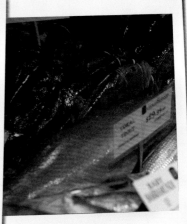

Brazilian Rice and Beans

Serves 4

Ingredients

For the rice

1 cup brown rice

1 tablespoon olive oil

½ onion, chopped

For the beans

2 cups dried black beans

1 onion, chopped

2 garlic cloves

1 tablespoon olive oil

sea salt and freshly ground black pepper

3 bay leaves

2 teaspoons Worcestershire sauce

Method

1. Rinse the rice under cold water. Heat the olive oil in a pan and brown the onion. Add the rice and 2 cups water to the pan and boil. Once boiled, reduce to simmer until all the water is absorbed and the rice is cooked. (If all the water has been absorbed, but the rice is not cooked, add a little more water.)

2. Place the black beans in a pressure cooker and add water to cover with an excess of approximately 1½in. Close the cooker and bring to a boil. Once it's boiled, reduce the heat to medium-low for approximately 20-25 minutes. The beans will be cooked once they are soft, but not mushy.

3. Brown the onion and garlic with the olive oil in another pan. Pour the beans from the pressure cooker into the pan with the salt, pepper, and bay leaves and let simmer for approximately 20 minutes. Add Worcestershire sauce to taste.

*top tip

White fish is very rich in B vitamins, which are good for increasing the metabolism and also improving your skin, cells, and immune system

Quinoa with Broiled Fish

Serves 4

Ingredients

2 tablespoons coconut oil

2 stems of purple sprouting broccoli, chopped

½ cup green beans, chopped

½ red bell pepper, chopped

½ yellow bell pepper, chopped

1 cup quinoa

zest of 1 lemon

1in piece of ginger, peeled and grated

4 fillets sea bream, red snapper, or sea bass

Method

1. Preheat the broiler.

2. Heat the coconut oil in a sauté pan over medium heat and cook the chopped vegetables until they are cooked but retain a slight crunch.

3. Cook the quinoa in another pan with 1¾ cups water until the water has evaporated and it's al dente. When the quinoa is ready, put it into the pan with the vegetables and mix it together. Keep warm.

4. Spread the lemon and ginger over the fish and broil for 8-10 minutes, turning halfway through.

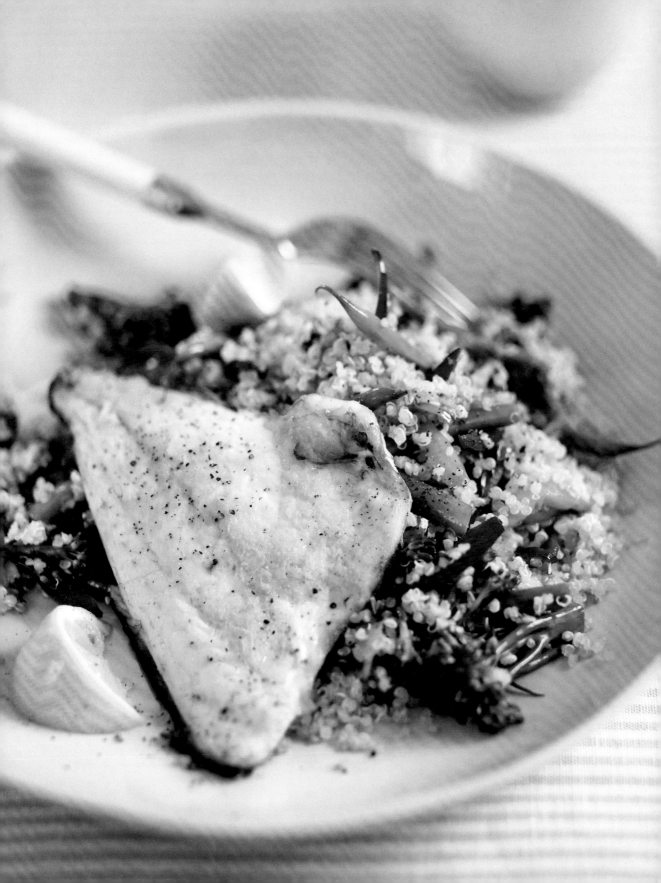

Salmon Sashimi
with Paperthin Salad

Serves 4

Ingredients
7oz boneless, skinless fresh salmon fillet
freshly ground black pepper

For the paperthin salad
2 baby carrots
2 baby zucchini
2 baby turnips
4 red radishes
2 baby beets
a bowl of iced water

For the dressing
1 cup jalapeño chiles, seeded and
finely chopped
½ tablespoon sea salt
1 garlic clove, chopped
⅓ cup rice vinegar
⅔ cup grapeseed oil

Method
1. Preheat a non-stick frying pan until medium-hot, season the salmon fillets with black pepper, then sear them for 5 seconds on each side. Make sure that all the outside has been completely seared and has turned white, then plunge them immediately into iced water to stop the cooking process. Drain and pat dry with paper towels, then refrigerate.

2. Prepare the salad, keeping the beets on the side. Slice the baby vegetables lengthwise very thinly on a mandolin grater into a bowl of iced water. Leave them in the iced water for 5 minutes to make them crunchy.

3. Repeat the same process with the beets, but place the slices in a separate bowl of iced water to keep the color from running into the other vegetables.

4. Drain the baby vegetables and the beets and then mix together.

5. Make up the jalapeño dressing by whisking together all the ingredients. Pour into the bottom of the serving dish, so that it completely covers the bottom.

6. Cut the chilled, seared salmon into slices about ⅛in thick and arrange across the center of the plate, then place the vegetable salad in the center on top of the salmon.

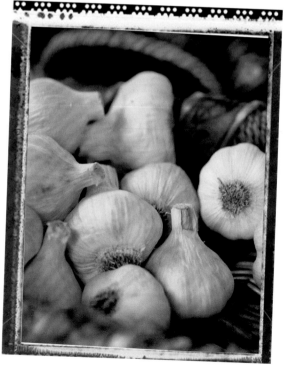

Fish Papillote

Serves 4

Ingredients

4 x 7oz monkfish fillets
5½oz mussels
3oz clams
juice of 1 lemon
1 onion, chopped
2 garlic cloves, sliced
a sprig of thyme
a small bunch of cilantro
⅓ cup fish stock
2½ tablespoons white wine
5½ tablespoons unsalted butter
sea salt and freshly ground black pepper,
to taste
¾ cup steamed rice, to serve

Method

1. Preheat the oven to 400°F.

2. Thinly slice the monkfish fillets.

3. Steam the mussels and clams in a little lemon juice and cover until they just start to open. Set aside.

4. Sauté the onion and garlic in half the butter until soft. Add the herbs and then remove from the heat.

5. Take 4 sheets of parchment paper and place some onion and herbs in the middle of each sheet along with the clams and mussels.

6. Lay the fish on top and pick up the edges of the paper so the stock and wine will not spill out. Pour in the stock, white wine, and remaining butter, then fold over the paper to form a parcel and staple shut.

7. Place on a hot baking sheet and cook in the preheated oven for 10-15 minutes. Once done, cut open the paper and serve with some steamed rice.

*top tip

Try to buy the freshest fish possible—
go to your local fishmonger and
ask what they have in that day

Portuguese Salt Cod

Serves 4

Ingredients

1 large onion, thinly sliced
1 red chile, thinly sliced
2 garlic cloves, thinly sliced
1 tablespoon olive oil
2 tablespoons tomato paste
1 teaspoon smoked paprika
2 tablespoons sherry or red wine vinegar
1 x 14oz can chopped tomatoes
1 x 14oz can cooked chickpeas
sea salt and freshly ground black pepper
14oz salt cod, soaked overnight, rinsed and drained twice
a bunch of parsley, chopped
extra virgin olive oil, for drizzling

Method

1. In a large pan, gently cook the onion, chile, and garlic in the olive oil until softened, then add the tomato paste and paprika and cook for another 3 minutes. Add the vinegar and simmer for 2-3 minutes. Add the tomatoes, chickpeas, and salt and pepper and bring to a steady simmer.

2. Add the salt cod and continue to gently simmer for roughly 15 minutes, until the cod is cooked and has started to flake.

3. Taste for seasoning and stir in the parsley.

4. Serve in pasta bowls with a drizzle of extra virgin olive oil and a green salad.

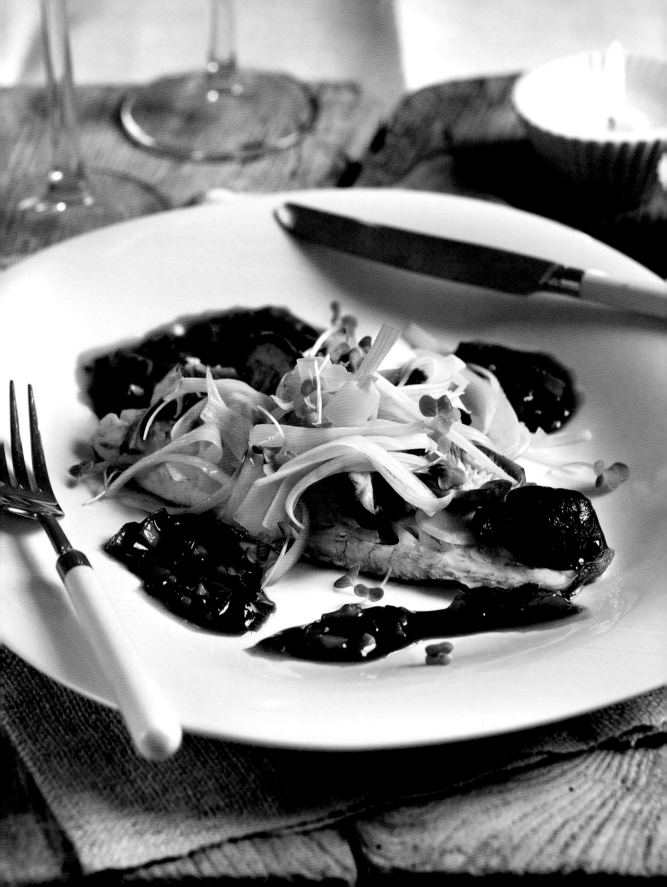

Cantonese Steamed Sea Bass with Shiitake Mushrooms, Leek, and Ginger

Serves 4

Ingredients

4 x 3½oz fillets sea bass
⅓ cup shiitake mushrooms, chopped
2in piece of ginger, thinly sliced
½ tablespoon vegetable oil
2 leeks, julienned
⅔ cup organic chicken stock
2 tablespoons oyster sauce
2 tablespoons soy sauce
2 tablespoons sesame oil
⅔ cup baby mustard cress

Method

1. Steam the fish for 7 minutes with half of the shiitake mushrooms on top.

2. Shallow fry the ginger in very hot vegetable oil for 3-4 minutes until golden and crisp, then drain on paper towels.

3. After 7 minutes, add the leek and deep-fried ginger to the fish and continue cooking for 3 minutes.

4. In a hot pan, reduce the chicken stock, oyster sauce, soy sauce, and the rest of the shiitake mushrooms until thick. Add the sesame oil.

5. Transfer the sea bass to a plate with some baby cress on top and pour the sauce around the fish.

*top tip
Sprinkle dried chili flakes onto your food. Studies show it can speed up your metabolism

Chicken Cassoulet

Serves 4

Ingredients

2 tablespoons olive oil
2 onions, peeled, halved, and sliced
6 garlic cloves, unpeeled
2 tablespoons tomato paste
2 bay leaves
½ cup white wine
2 carrots, peeled and sliced into ¾in rounds
2 x 14oz cans chopped tomatoes
sea salt and freshly ground black pepper
8 chicken thighs and/or drumsticks
2 x 14oz cans navy beans
a small bunch of parsley, finely chopped

Method

1. Preheat the oven to 350°F.

2. Heat the olive oil in a large sauté pan and cook the onions and garlic over low heat.

3. After 7 minutes, add the tomato paste and bay leaves and cook for 5 minutes, then add the wine and simmer to reduce a little.

4. Add the carrots and canned tomatoes and a pinch of salt and pepper. Bring to a simmer and turn off the heat.

5. Place the chicken and navy beans in a large dutch oven and pour the tomato sauce over the top. Bake in the oven for 1-1½ hours until the chicken is falling off the bone.

6. Scatter the parsley over the top and enjoy with a green salad.

Thai Shrimp and Coconut Broth

Serves 4

Ingredients
1 tablespoon vegetable oil
a bunch of scallions, finely sliced
1 green chile, finely sliced
1 medium piece of fresh ginger, peeled and grated
1 tablespoon red Thai curry paste
4 kaffir lime leaves
1 x 9oz block creamed coconut
1 quart organic vegetable stock
4 tablespoons tamari soy sauce
4 tablespoons fish sauce
1 cup bean sprouts
2 heads bok choy, chopped
1 cup cooked shrimp
⅔ cup cooked rice noodles

To garnish
a bunch of cilantro, chopped
1 lime, quartered

Method
1. In a large, deep pan, heat the oil and gently cook the scallions, chile, and ginger.

2. Once softened, add the curry paste and lime leaves. After a couple of minutes, add the coconut and stock. Bring to a simmer and add the soy sauce and fish sauce. Add the bean sprouts, bok choy, and shrimp and continue to simmer for another 8–10 minutes.

3. Divide the rice noodles between 4 soup bowls and ladle over the broth. Garnish with the chopped cilantro and lime wedges.

Sesame Salmon Tataki

Serves 4

Ingredients
2 tablespoons olive oil
10½oz fresh salmon fillets
a pinch of sea salt
⅓ cup white sesame seeds, toasted
1¼ cups carrots, julienned
½ cucumber, julienned
5 white radishes, thinly sliced
5 red radishes, thinly sliced
¾oz seaweed (nori sheet)
finely grated zest of 1 lime
a small bunch of cilantro, chopped
sea salt and freshly ground black pepper, to taste

For the ponzu jalapeño dressing
⅓ cup jalapeño chiles, seeded and chopped
1 teaspoon sea salt
2 teaspoons garlic, chopped
¾ cup rice vinegar
1 cup grapeseed oil

Method
1. Place a non-stick pan over medium heat and add 2 tablespoons oil. Season the salmon with salt and crust with sesame seeds. When the oil is hot, sear the salmon sesame-side down and cook for 4–8 minutes. Remove the salmon from the pan, set aside, and slice on an angle.

2. To make the dressing, mix all the ingredients together in a small bowl.

3. Divide the carrots, cucumber, radish, and seaweed between 4 plates. Top with the sliced salmon, sprinkle with the lime zest and cilantro, season to taste, and serve with ponzu jalapeño dressing.

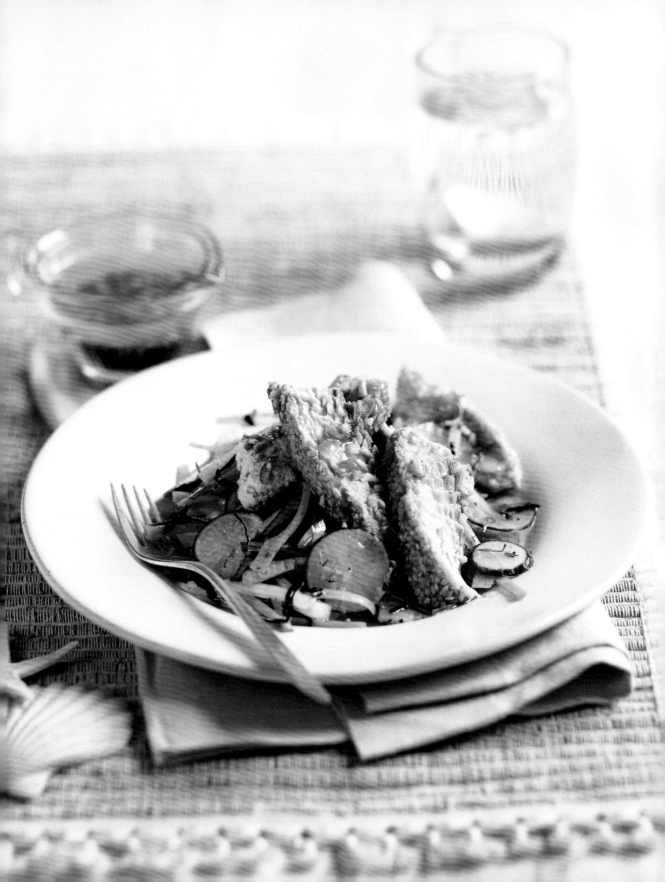

*top tip

Be adventurous with fish! Head to your local fishmonger and try out ones you've never had before. Don't get stuck in a cod or salmon rut!

Grouper Ceviche

Serves 4

Ingredients

4 x 5½oz grouper fillets
juice of ½ grapefruit
juice of 4 limes
¼ teaspoon chopped Scotch Bonnet chile
1 teaspoon sea salt
1 cup red bell pepper, diced
¾ red onion, diced
1 cup tomatoes, diced
1½ tablespoons olive oil
⅓ cup finely diced black olives
a large bunch of cilantro, leaves picked and chopped
¼ cup scallions, white parts only, chopped
2 avocados, halved
lemon, cut into segments, to serve
a pinch of sumac, for dusting

Method

1. Cut the grouper into ¼-in thick bite-sized pieces.

2. In a bowl, combine the grapefruit juice, lime juice, and Scotch bonnet. Add the fish and marinate, covered, for about 10 minutes.

3. Drain the fish in a strainer and discard the marinade. While the fish is still in the strainer, salt it evenly. Transfer the fish to a bowl, add the next ingredients up to the avocado, and stir well.

4. Place the avocado in the center of the plate with the ceviche on top. Serve with lemon segments and finish with a dusting of sumac.

Fish Tacos

Serves 4

Ingredients

1 large jicama or turnip (for 12 Taco-shapes slices and ¾ cup for the sauce)
⅔ cup low-fat plain yogurt
¼ cup serrano chiles (stem and seeds removed), finely chopped
a small bunch of cilantro, leaves picked and chopped
1 teaspoon sea salt, plus more for seasoning
2 tablespoons lime juice
½ red onion, thinly sliced
12 x 2½oz sea bass fillet strips, skin off (or use haddock, cod, or tilapia)
1½ tablespoons extra virgin olive oil
1 lime, cut into wedges, to serve

Method

1. Peel the jicama and slice thinly into taco shapes. Reserve ¾ cup jicama scraps for the yogurt sauce.

2. Purée the yogurt, serrano chile, cilantro leaves, and jicama scraps to a smooth sauce and season with the salt.

3. In a small pan, bring the lime juice to a boil and cook the red onion until glazed.

4. Season the fish with more salt and broil under a hot broiler for 3–4 minutes on each side.

5. Place the fish on the jicama tacos and drizzle with olive oil. Add the red onion slices and the spicy cilantro yogurt. Serve garnished with lime wedges.

Kashmiri Chicken and Yogurt Curry

Serves 4

Ingredients

1 tablespoon olive oil
8 deboned and skinless chicken thighs, cut into thick strips
1 large onion, thinly sliced
2 garlic cloves, finely chopped
1 large piece of fresh ginger, peeled and grated
1 green chile, thinly sliced
a bunch of cilantro, roots and leaves separated and finely chopped
1 teaspoon ground coriander
1 teaspoon ground cardamom
1 teaspoon turmeric
1 cup sliced almonds
⅓ cup organic chicken stock
1 cup plain yogurt
sea salt and freshly ground black pepper
1 cup brown rice, cooked

Method

1. In a large, heavy-bottomed pan, heat the oil and quickly brown the chicken. Transfer to a plate and set aside.

2. Add the onion, garlic, ginger, chile, and cilantro roots to the pan and cook for approximately 10 minutes, until softened. Add the spices and cook for another 5 minutes, stirring frequently. Add the almond slices and then the chicken. Stir well and add the stock and yogurt, salt, and pepper. Cook over medium heat, at a gentle simmer for 35–45 minutes.

3. Taste for seasoning before serving with brown rice and the cilantro leaves sprinkled over the top.

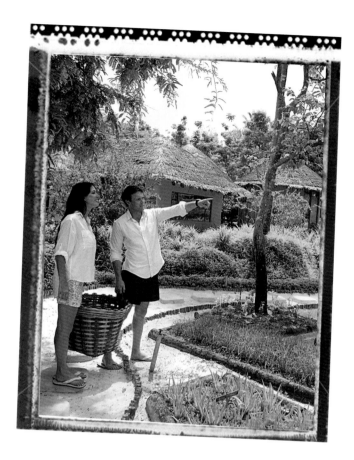

*top tip

Try this with other meats, such as lamb, beef, or fish. It tastes fantastic with shrimp. Remember to vary your cooking times according to the type of protein you use

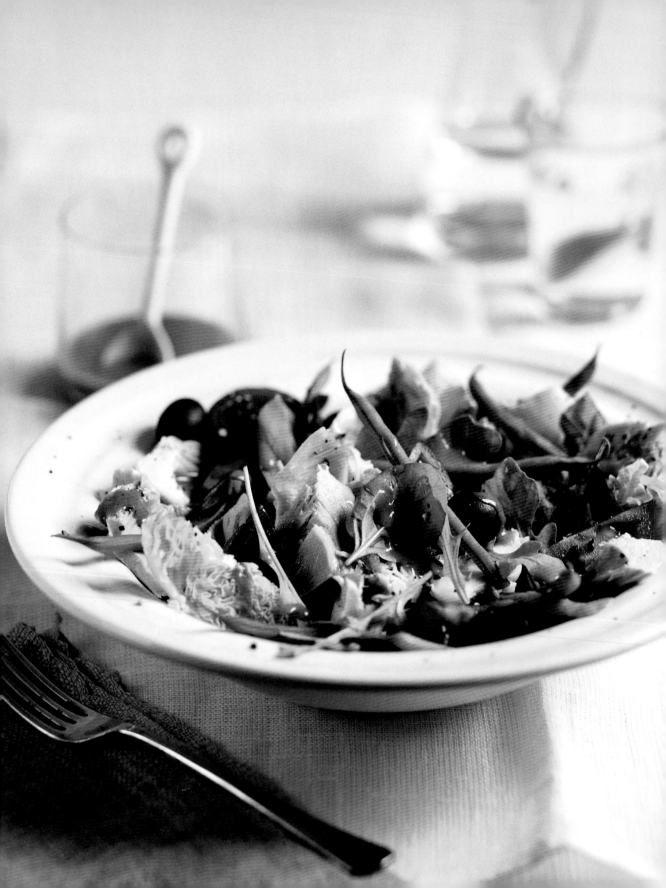

French Niçoise Salad

Serves 4

Ingredients

2 cups green beans
4 cups mixed green lettuce leaves
4 cooked artichoke hearts, halved
4 plum tomatoes, cut into wedges
¾ cup black pitted olives
7oz fresh tuna, cooked and flaked

For the dressing

2 teaspoons Dijon mustard
⅓ cup olive oil
1 garlic clove, crushed
2 teaspoons balsamic vinegar

Method

1. Steam the green beans. Mix all the remaining salad ingredients together in a bowl. Mix all the dressing ingredients together in a separate bowl, then drizzle the dressing over the salad and serve.

Mexican Black Bean Chili

Serves 4

Ingredients

1 tablespoon olive oil
1 red onion, chopped
1 garlic clove, finely chopped
1 red chile, thinly sliced
1 teaspoon chile powder
1 teaspoon ground cumin
1 teaspoon paprika
2 tablespoons tomato paste
1 carrot, sliced
1 red, yellow, or orange bell pepper, cut into strips
1 x 14oz can black or kidney beans
1 x 14oz can chopped tomatoes
sea salt and freshly ground black pepper

To serve

1 lime, quartered
plain yogurt
a small bunch of cilantro, finely chopped
jalapeño peppers, chopped, to garnish

Method

1. In a large pan, heat the oil and gently cook the onion, garlic, and chile for about 10 minutes. Once they are softened, add the spices and cook for 5 minutes. Add the tomato paste and cook for 3–4 minutes.

2. Add the carrot, bell pepper, beans, chopped tomatoes, and salt and pepper and simmer over medium heat for 30 minutes.

3. Serve with lime wedges, a spoonful of yogurt, and the chopped cilantro on top. Garnish with the jalapeño peppers.

*it's easy

When you make a salad, make a big batch and have it for lunch the next day in a lettuce wrap

Conch Salad

Serves 5

Ingredients

1lb fresh conch meat (or crab or shrimp)

1 large onion

1½ green bell peppers

3 celery ribs

1 cucumber

4 tomatoes

1 tablespoon vinegar

2 tablespoons olive oil

juice of 2 lemons

juice of 2 oranges

½ teaspoon sea salt

¼ teaspoon freshly ground black pepper

Method

1. Chop the conch and vegetables into ½–¾in pieces and combine with the vinegar, olive oil, and lemon and orange juice.

2. Add the salt and pepper. Taste and adjust the seasoning. Keep refrigerated. Conch salad always tastes better on the second day.

*top tip

Don't overcook your steak as rare or medium-rare steak is the most flavorful and it'll satisfy your tastebuds for longer

My top steaks

I have traveled far and wide and spent years researching all of the most celebrated steak houses and the undisputed No.1 steak in the world—by a long, long way—is the wagyu sirloin steak at the **Rockpool Bar and Grill** in Sydney. The chef, Neil Perry, is a genius. Then, and in no particular order as these are all as good as each other, **Mastro's Steak Houses** in the US, **JW's Steak House** in London (which also serves the best cheesecake in the world, for a cheat day) and **Cut** in Beverly Hills for an incredible porterhouse.

Grilled Rib Eye Steak

Serves 4

Ingredients

4 x 6oz rib eye steaks

1 tablespoon olive oil

2 large handfuls of arugula

20 cherry tomatoes

a pinch of sea salt

a pinch of freshly ground black pepper

extra virgin olive oil, for drizzling

aged balsamic vinegar, for drizzling

Method

1. Preheat a grill pan until very hot. Season the steaks, rub in the olive oil, and grill for 3–4 minutes per side, according to taste.

2. Wash and clean the arugula leaves and halve the cherry tomatoes. Season both with salt and pepper and drizzle with olive oil.

3. When the meat is cooked, transfer to a plate, topping it with the arugula and cherry tomatoes. Drizzle some oil and aged balsamic vinegar on top of the salad.

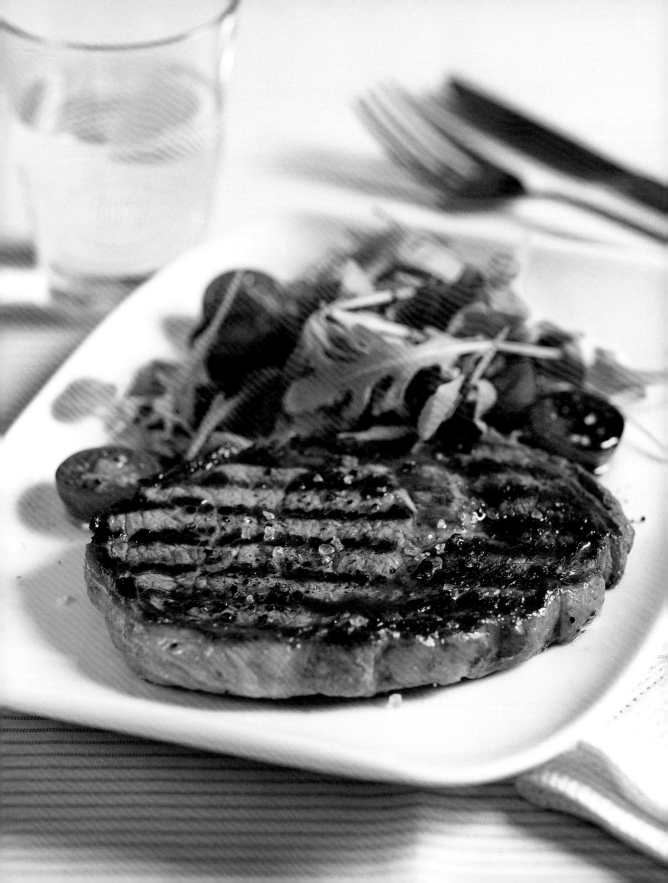

HERE'S MY HANDY "BAD, BETTER & BEST"

BAD	BETTER	BEST
Bad: Deep-fried turkey burger with fries **Why?** Full of trans fats, which lower good cholesterol and raise bad cholesterol	**Better:** Grilled turkey fillet with butternut squash **Why?** No trans fats and full of vitamins and nutrients	**Best:** Turkey breast on a bed of spinach, avocado, and tomatoes **Why?** A great source of clean, organic, lean protein and a perfectly balanced meal of protein, fats, and carbohydrates
Bad: Lamb doner kebab with creamy garlic sauce on white pita bread **Why?** Full of flour and sugar	**Better:** Shoulder of lamb with rosemary and garlic cloves **Why?** Garlic is a great immune system booster	**Best:** Organic lamb steak with peas **Why?** Organic meat is hormone-free and peas are packed with healthy fiber
Bad: Flour tortilla wrap with fried chicken and sour cream **Why?** Packed full of added salt and sugar	**Better:** Whole wheat wrap with freshly diced chicken and tomato salsa **Why?** A good source of fiber, protein, and nutrients	**Best:** Lettuce wrap with organic sliced chicken and freshly made guacamole **Why?** A great source of nutrients and guacamole is loaded with healthy omega fatty acids
Bad: Fish and chips with creamy tartar sauce **Why?** Full of trans fat	**Better:** Homemade fishfingers with a breadcrumb crust **Why?** Much healthier than shop-bought, especially when oven-baked	**Best:** Whole baked sea bass **Why?** Sea bass is a great source of omega 3 fatty acids (a natural anti-inflammatory)
Bad: Battered non-organic chicken in a white bun with bbq sauce **Why?** A salt, sugar, and flour cocktail	**Better:** Barbecued chicken breast with wild rice and tomato salsa **Why?** Full of nutrients and amino acids, plus wild rice is a slower releasing carbohydrate	**Best:** Broiled organic chicken and radicchio salad **Why?** A light, clean, organic meal and packed with antioxidants as radicchio is a healthy superfood
Bad: Non-organic, frozen, bread crumbed burger with deep-fried potato wedges **Why?** Bread crumbs can be inflammatory to your digestive system	**Better:** Homemade ground beef patty with fresh cut potato chips **Why?** Homemade beef patties can be made minus the bread crumbs and salt, which is better for your health	**Best:** Grass-fed, organic beef patties with sautéed mushrooms and sweet potato **Why?** A source of iron and carnitine, which is great for increasing energy levels

WORLD CUISINE GUIDE:

BAD	BETTER	BEST
Bad: Pasta with creamy sauce **Why?** No protein or fiber content	**Better:** Whole-grain pasta with shrimp **Why?** Contains fiber and protein to help keep you feeling full	**Best:** White miso scallops **Why?** A yummy, meaty fish. Full of essential fatty acids
Bad: Tuna sushi rolls with almost no tuna, mostly rice and mayonnaise **Why?** Very low nutrient content	**Better:** Tuna sushi rolls made with brown rice **Why?** A great balance of fats, protein, and carbohydrates	**Best:** Tuna sashimi with a seaweed salad **Why?** Seaweed has cancer-protecting properties
Bad: Packaged seafood paella **Why?** Loaded with salt	**Better:** Homemade seafood paella with brown rice **Why?** Full of essential fatty acids	**Best:** Rock oysters **Why?** A rich source of zinc
Bad: Deep-fried calamari with ketchup **Why?** Very high in trans fats	**Better:** Broiled calamari with tartar sauce **Why?** Squid boosts your immune system and stabilizes blood sugar levels	**Best:** Broiled squid on a bed of kale **Why?** All the benefits (see left), plus kale helps your body to detoxify
Bad: Greasy fried lamb in a white bread roll **Why?** Fatty and full of flour	**Better:** Shredded lamb on a spit with hummus and rice **Why?** Full of flavor and without the flour	**Best:** Broiled lamb cutlets with chermoula dip and roasted vegetables **Why?** A good balance of fiber and protein to keep you feeling full
Bad: Fish pie with a lot of crust and mashed potatoes **Why?** Full of flour	**Better:** Salmon fillet in a tomato and basil sauce **Why?** Tomatoes have excellent anti-inflammatory properties	**Best:** Oven-poached organic salmon **Why?** Full of omega-3 fatty acids
Bad: Shrimp tempura with rice and sweet and sour sauce **Why?** High trans fat content and sugar	**Better:** Shrimp pad thai with rice noodles **Why?** Rice noodles are low GI so release energy slowly	**Best:** Lemongrass and coconut shrimp with glass noodles **Why?** A balance of fats, protein, and carbohydrates

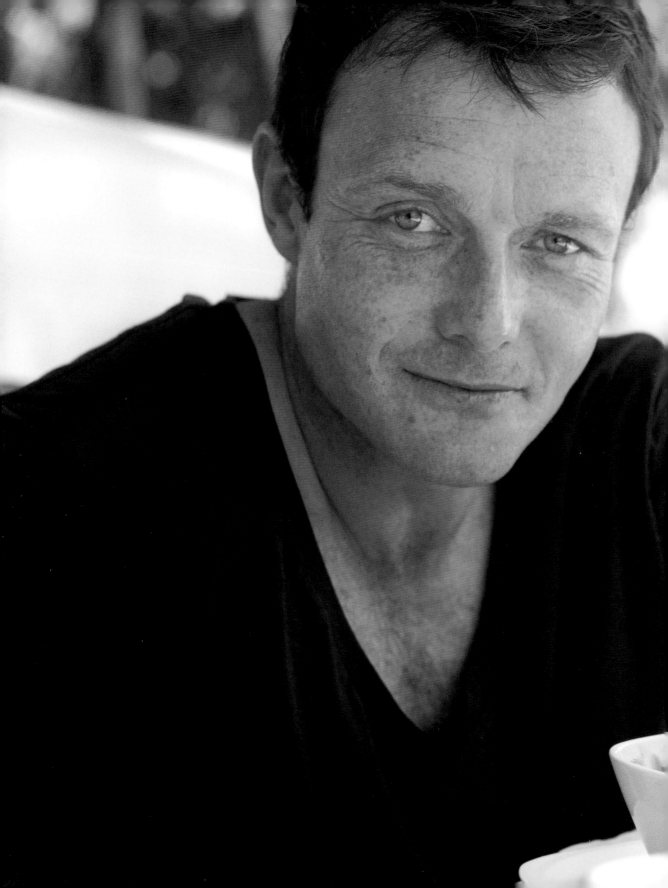

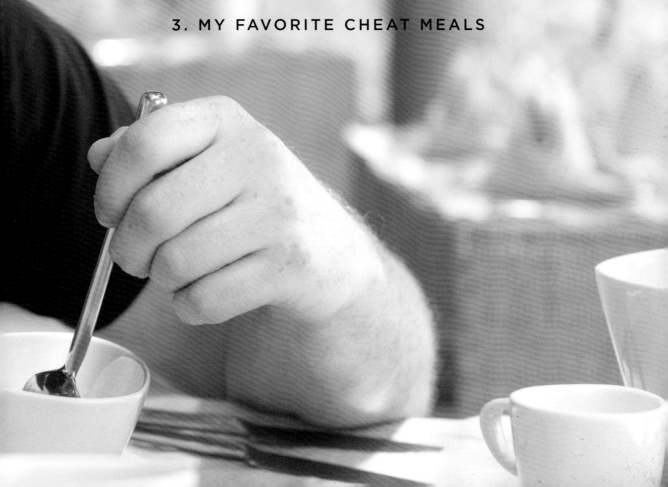

CHAPTER 7

CLEAN AND LEAN CHEATS AND TREATS

THIS CHAPTER WILL REVEAL:

1. THE BODY BENEFITS OF CHOCOLATE CAKE (YES, REALLY!)

2. WHY YOUR BODY NEEDS A TREAT

3. MY FAVORITE CHEAT MEALS

In my first book, *The Clean & Lean Diet*, I introduced readers to the concept of a "cheat meal." Basically, it can be whatever you want it to be—chocolate, a plate of ribs, some creamy pasta, fudge, ice cream ... anything—and I tell all my clients to have one a week.

The idea behind the cheat meal is that your metabolism gets such a shock from the huge and unexpected amount of calories and fat, it revs up a notch and becomes even better at burning fat. Of course, if you eat cheat meals all the time, this doesn't happen because it isn't a shock to your metabolism.

The second benefit of having a cheat meal is that it keeps you from becoming bored. If you eat Clean & Lean 90 percent of the time, having the odd treat keeps things fun and prevents you from craving the bad stuff.

So this chapter is made up of all my favorite cheat meals, including my wedding cake.

QUICK TIPS FOR A CHEAT MEAL

Here is my cheat meal advice:

Choose your treat wisely...

✳ Don't go for something pre-packaged, stuffed full of additives, and that tastes bland. If you're going to treat yourself, have something delicious. As a rule, homemade cakes, cookies, and brownies taste better than packaged ones full of preservatives. The same goes for other meals—pasta with a rich, homemade creamy dressing tastes far better than a pre-made meal. If you're going to be bad, make it good!

Say goodbye to guilt...

✳ When you do have it, have it guilt-free. A cheat meal is pointless if you stuff it down quickly while feeling bad or ashamed. So many of us grab our favorite food—like a chocolate bar—and eat it while we're walking along the road, on the bus, or driving our car. But what's the point in that? You'll barely taste it after the first mouthful because you'll be in a hurry and concentrating on something else. Instead, savor your cheat meal. Sit down and eat it slowly, enjoying every mouthful.

Don't binge...

✳ In theory, it's fine to have as much as you like of your cheat meal, but don't eat so much of something it leaves you feel disgustingly full and bloated. That isn't a treat. Eat as much as you like, but stop well before your stomach starts to hurt and you feel sick.

Eat slowly...

✳ When I used to have my cheat meal, I would wolf it down. It was like I was trying to eat it all up before anybody saw me. But that isn't how a cheat meal should be eaten. Instead, you should eat it "mindfully," and that means slowly. Chew it properly, take in the flavors, savor each bite, breathe, and enjoy it.

Eat it well before bedtime...

✳ Don't eat a lot of sugar and/or chocolate too close to bedtime. Both sugar and chocolate—which contains caffeine—are stimulants and they can disrupt your sleep. So try to have your cheat meal well before it's time to go to sleep.

*top tip

Listen to your body... if your cheat meal leaves you feeling bloated and gassy, try something else. Remember, your body is your own nutritionist and it will tell you what it can and can't handle

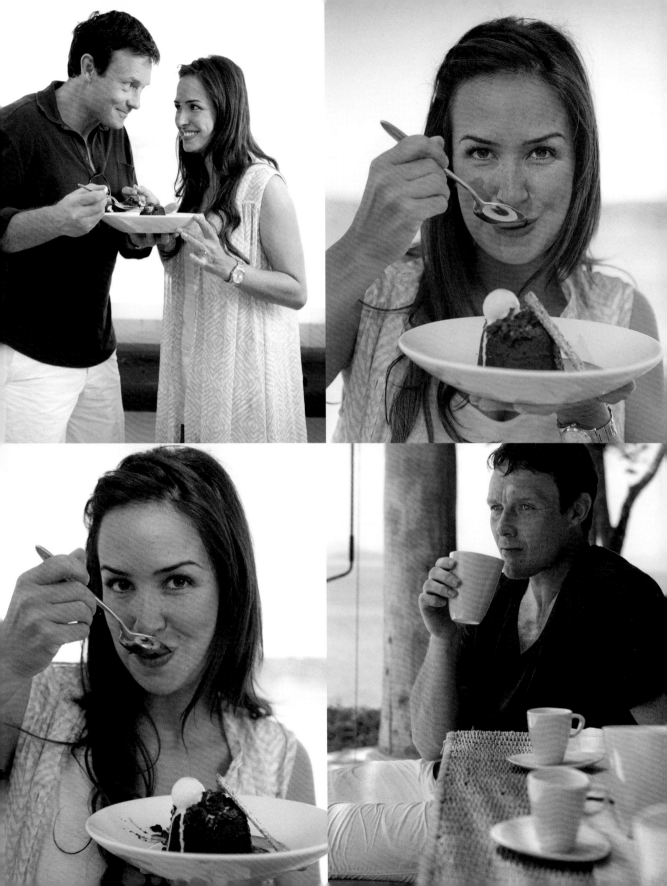

*Our wedding was full of so
many beautiful moments and
memories... celebrating with the
people we love, eating good food,
and dancing badly (at least I was
dancing badly). We also had our
favorite dessert in the world—
Clara's peanut butter chocolate
cake! It's just so good for so many
reasons and it will always bring
back memories of the happiest
moment in my life, ever*

James and Christiane's Wedding Cake (Chocolate Cake with Peanut Butter Frosting)

Serves 8-10

Ingredients
¾ cup cocoa powder
2¼ cups all-purpose flour
2½ cups sugar
2 teaspoons baking soda
1 teaspoon sea salt
1 cup vegetable oil
1 cup sour cream
1½ cups water
2 teaspoons white wine vinegar
1 teaspoon vanilla extract
2 organic eggs

For the frosting
½ cup + 1 tablespoon softened butter
1 cup cream cheese
5½ cups confectioners' sugar
⅔ cup smooth peanut butter

Method
1. Preheat the oven to 300°F.

2. Mix together the cocoa, flour, sugar, baking soda, and salt. Add the oil and sour cream, all the while whisking together. Gradually add the water, followed by the vinegar and vanilla extract. Finally, add the eggs.

3. Grease 2 x 9-inch round cake pans and divide the mixture between them. Bake in the preheated oven for 30–35 minutes. Let cool.

4. To make the frosting, beat the butter until smooth. Add the cream cheese and beat. Gradually sift in the confectioners' sugar. Add the peanut butter and beat again. Ice the cooled cakes and place one on top of the other.

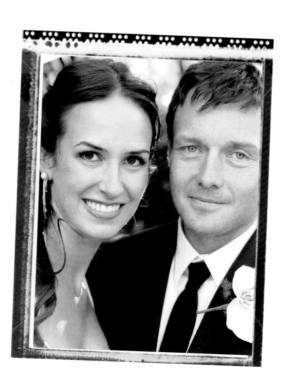

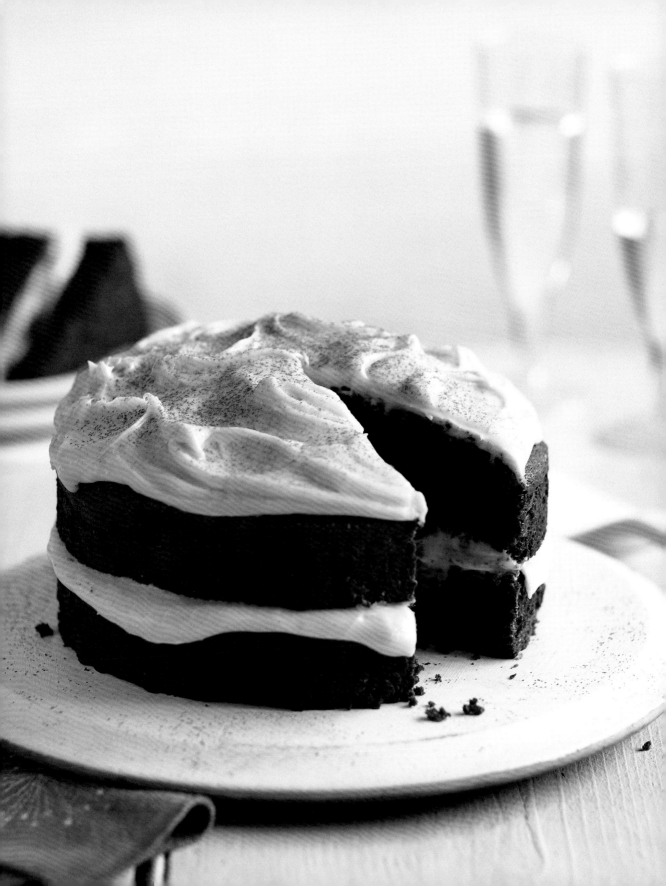

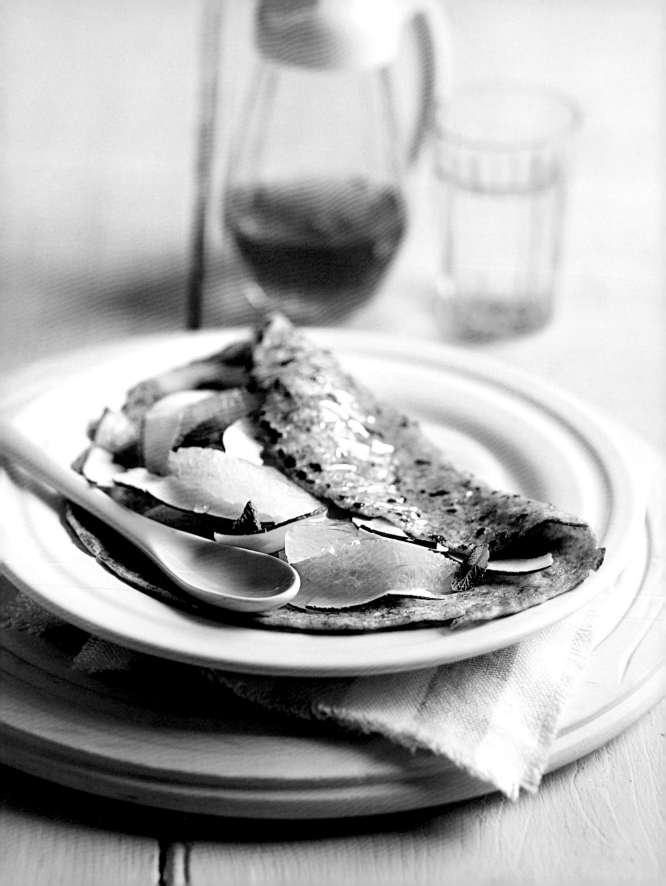

Coconut Crêpes, Agave Syrup, and Grapefruit

Serves 4

Ingredients

1 cup coconut milk
1½ tablespoons grapefruit juice
a large pinch of grapefruit zest
a pinch of salt
1½ tablespoons agave syrup, plus extra
for drizzling
2 organic egg whites, beaten
1 cup whole wheat flour
2 tablespoons shredded coconut
1 tablespoon coconut oil
1 grapefruit, peeled and cut into segments
4½oz young coconut flesh, in strips
sprig of mint, leaves removed

Method

1. Mix the coconut milk with the grapefruit juice and zest, salt, and the 1½ tablespoons agave syrup.

2. Beat the egg whites, then fold them into the grapefruit mixture. Slowly add the flour and the coconut.

3. Heat a frying pan over medium heat and add the oil. Wipe the pan for excess oil with a piece of paper towel and pour in 1 small ladleful of batter, 2 if there's room, and cook for 3–4 minutes on each side, until the batter turns golden. Between crêpes, wipe the pan with the oiled paper towel.

4. Top each crêpe with the grapefruit segments and the coconut strips. Serve with the agave syrup drizzled over the top and decorate with mint leaves.

Naughty-But-Nice Cheesecake

Serves 8

Ingredients

2 cups graham crackers
1¼ cups rolled oats
½ cup + 2 tablespoons unsalted butter, cubed
2½ cups cream cheese
1 vanilla bean or pure vanilla essence
¾ cup superfine sugar
zest of 1 lemon
zest of 1 orange
1¼ cups heavy cream

To serve

1 pint organic blueberries, strawberries, or raspberries
sugar, to taste

Method

1. Crush the graham crackers. In a pan, heat the oats over low heat until darker in color, then add the cubed butter and the crushed graham crackers. Stir until combined. Remove from the heat and spoon into a loose-bottomed pan, flatten, and refrigerate for 1 hour.

2. Place the cream cheese, vanilla, sugar, and lemon and orange zest in a blender and mix until smooth.

3. Whisk the cream then gradually fold into the cream cheese mixture. Spoon the mixture evenly over the chilled crust. Refrigerate for 1 hour.

4. Squash the berries together to make them slightly liquidy, mix in a little sugar, then pour over the top of the cheesecake and serve.

Chocolate and Raspberry Molten Cake

Serves 4

Ingredients

¾ cup + 2 tablespoons unsalted butter
7oz good-quality dark chocolate, minimum 70 percent cocoa solids
½ cup sugar
4 large organic eggs, separated
1⅔ cups raspberries
¼ cup all-purpose flour
plain organic yogurt, to serve

Method

1. Preheat the oven to 400°F. Grease either 1 large round ovenproof dish or 4 individual ramekins.

2. Place the butter and chocolate in a pan and gently heat until melted. Remove from the heat, then add the sugar. Stir well. Add the egg yolks and stir well. Mash the raspberries and stir into the chocolate mixture with the flour.

3. Whisk the egg whites until stiff peaks form and fold into the chocolate, making sure the mixture is well combined. Pour into the prepared dish or ramekins and bake in the preheated oven for 15 minutes, or until they have just a slight wobble in the middle.

4. Serve with plain yogurt.

*top tip

This is a great cupcake recipe because they're easy to make and a teensy bit healthy. You can also vary the frosting flavors by adding caramel or dulce de leche instead of vanilla

The Cupcake Company's Banana Cupcake

Makes 12

Ingredients

1½ cups all-purpose flour
½ teaspoon baking powder
a pinch of freshly grated nutmeg
a pinch of sea salt
1 cup demerara sugar
½ cup + 1 tablespoon unsalted butter, melted and slightly cooled
2 organic eggs, lightly beaten
½ teaspoon vanilla extract
¼ cup milk
3 large, very ripe bananas, mashed

For the frosting

1 cup + 1 tablespoon unsalted butter, softened
5 cups confectioners' sugar, sifted
1 teaspoon vanilla extract
1 tablespoon milk

Method

1. Preheat the oven to 325°F.

2. In a large bowl, sift together the flour, baking powder, nutmeg, and salt. Stir in the sugar.

3. In a separate bowl mix together the butter, eggs, vanilla, milk, and mashed bananas. Add the dry ingredients and gently mix together.

4. Fill the cupcake liners three-quarters full and arrange on a baking sheet. Bake for approximately 25 minutes, until the cakes spring back to the touch (or a skewer inserted in the center comes out clean).

5. After 5 minutes, transfer the cupcakes onto a wire rack and cool.

6. Mix together all the frosting ingredients in a food processor until smooth. Spread over the top of the cupcakes and decorate how you like.

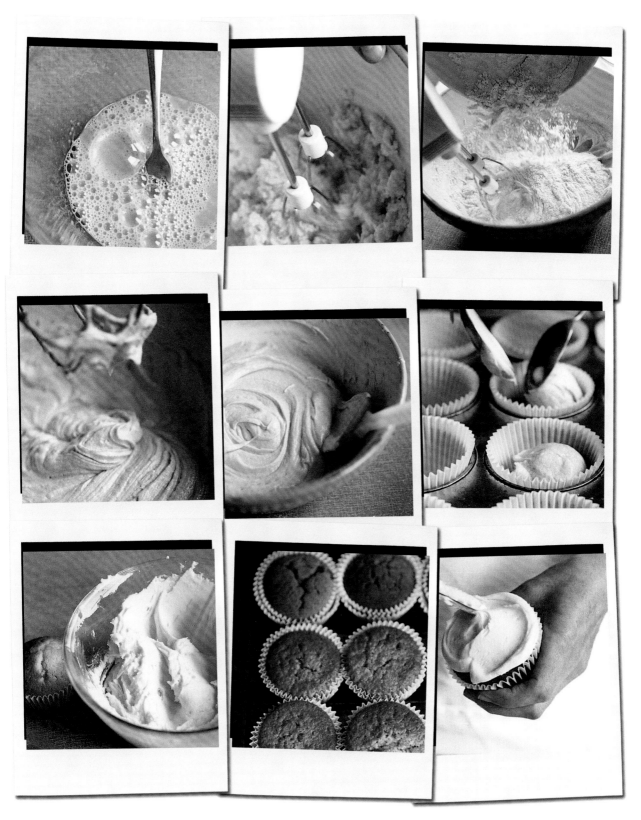

Vanilla Mascarpone with Toasted Coconut and Grated Chocolate and Raspberries

Serves 4

Ingredients
9oz mascarpone
1 vanilla bean, halved and seeds scraped out
1 cup shredded coconut, toasted until golden
1⅔ cups raspberries
3½oz good-quality dark chocolate, minimum 70 percent cocoa solids

Method
1. In a bowl, beat the mascarpone with the seeds from the vanilla bean. Mix in the coconut and the raspberries.

2. Divide the mixture between 4 serving bowls and grate the chocolate over the top.

Berry Blitz

Serves 6

Ingredients
1 pint blueberries
1 pint strawberries
1 pint raspberries
1 pint blackberries
1¼ cups plain yogurt
1 cup sliced almonds
a sprinkle of cinnamon

Method
Place all the berries in a serving bowl. Serve with a dollop of plain yogurt and a sprinkling of almonds and cinnamon on top.

*top tip
Berries are a great accompaniment to cheat meals. They taste sweet, so satisfy a sugar craving, yet they're full of vitamins and nutrients

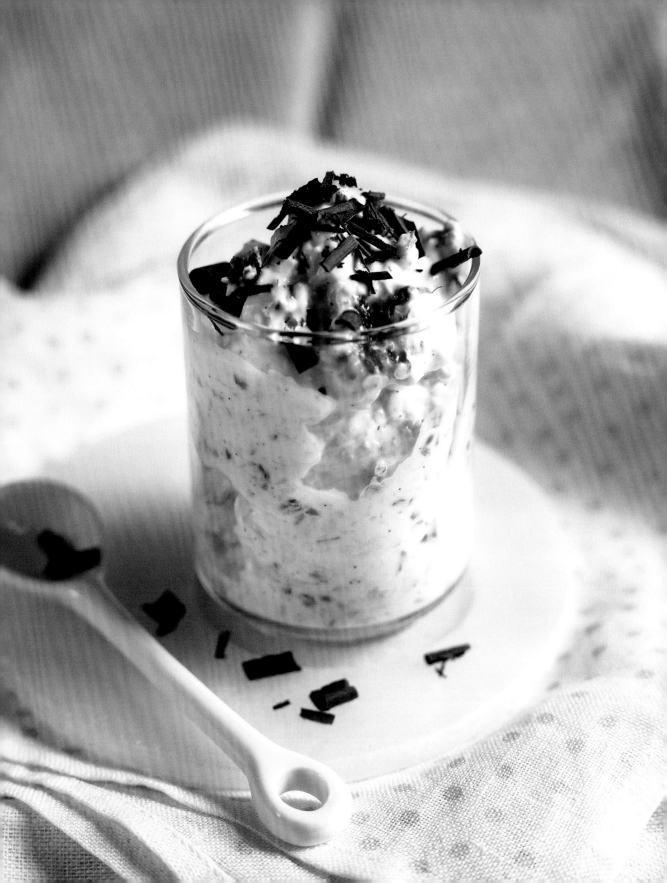

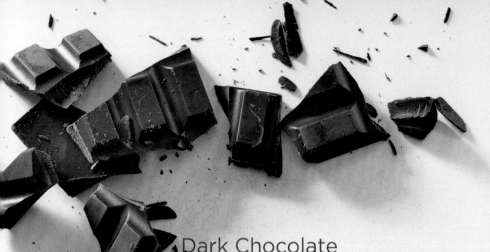

Dark Chocolate Fondant with Green Tea Ice Cream

Serves 4

Ingredients

For the green tea ice cream
½ cup heavy cream
½oz glucose powder
2 tablespoons powdered milk
1¼ tablespoons matcha powder (green tea)
¾ cup + 1 tablespoon milk
3 large organic egg yolks
¼ cup superfine sugar

For the chocolate fondant
4½oz good-quality dark chocolate
(70 percent cocoa solids)
½ cup + 1 tablespoon unsalted butter
2 organic eggs
2 large organic egg yolks
¼ cup superfine sugar
1½ tablespoons rice flour
extra rice flour, for dusting

Method

1. First make the ice cream. Combine all the ingredients except the egg yolks and sugar and bring to a gentle simmer, stirring occasionally. Whisk the egg yolks and sugar together. Add the hot green tea mixture to the egg yolks, one spoonful at a time, whisking continuously. Once all the ingredients are mixed well, strain the mixture and let cool before refrigerating overnight.

2. Churn the ice cream for 10 minutes, then place in the freezer.

3. Preheat the oven to 350°F. Grease 4 ring molds (no bigger than 3in in diameter and 2in in height) and dust them with flour. Cut square pieces of parchment paper (bigger than the rings) to place underneath.

4. Melt the chocolate and butter over a double boiler.

5. Whisk the whole eggs, yolks, and sugar to form a sabayon. Add the chocolate mixture and rice flour to the sabayon and mix until incorporated. Pour the mixture into a piping bag and fill molds to three quarters full. Bake in the preheated oven for 10 minutes.

6. Serve the chocolate fondants hot with the green tea ice cream.

*top tip
Green tea tea bags can be used when infused to the milk mixture, but the flavor and color will not be as intense.

Pistachio and Olive Oil Cake with Apple Sorbet

Serves 8–10

Ingredients
For the cake
¼ cup polenta
2 cups ground pistachios
⅓ cup all-purpose flour
1 teaspoon baking powder
½ cup olive oil
7 tablespoons unsalted butter, melted and cooled
3 organic eggs
1 cup superfine sugar
juice and zest of 1 lemon
juice of 1 orange
confectioners' sugar, for dusting

For the apple sorbet
3¼ cups apples, quartered
¾ cup superfine sugar
¼ cup glucose
¾ cup + 1 tablespoon water
2 tablespoons lemon juice

Method

1. Preheat the oven to 325 °F. Grease and line a 9in cake pan.

2. Mix the polenta, ground pistachios, flour, and baking powder together. Add the olive oil to the melted butter. Whisk the eggs and superfine sugar together until pale, then slowly whisk in the oil and butter. Whisk in the pistachio mixture, then add the lemon juice and zest and orange juice.

3. Transfer the cake mixture to the prepared pan and bake in the preheated oven for 40 minutes. The cake should be slightly underdone in the middle, so that if you insert a skewer it will come out with a little of the mixture sticking to it; leave for 10 minutes to cool in the pan, which will finish it off.

4. To make the sorbet, place the apples in the freezer for 2 hours. Place the sugar, glucose, and water in a pan and bring to a boil, stirring until the sugar has dissolved.

5. Remove the apples from the freezer and place in a blender or food processor along with the syrup. Add the lemon juice, blend, then pass through a fine sieve. Transfer the mixture to an ice-cream maker.

7. Serve the cake with a dusting of sugar and a scoop of sorbet—delicious!

*top tip

Go for the best-quality dark chocolate you can afford. It will contain more health-boosting antioxidants and will taste better, meaning a little bit will go a long way when it comes to satisfying a sweet craving

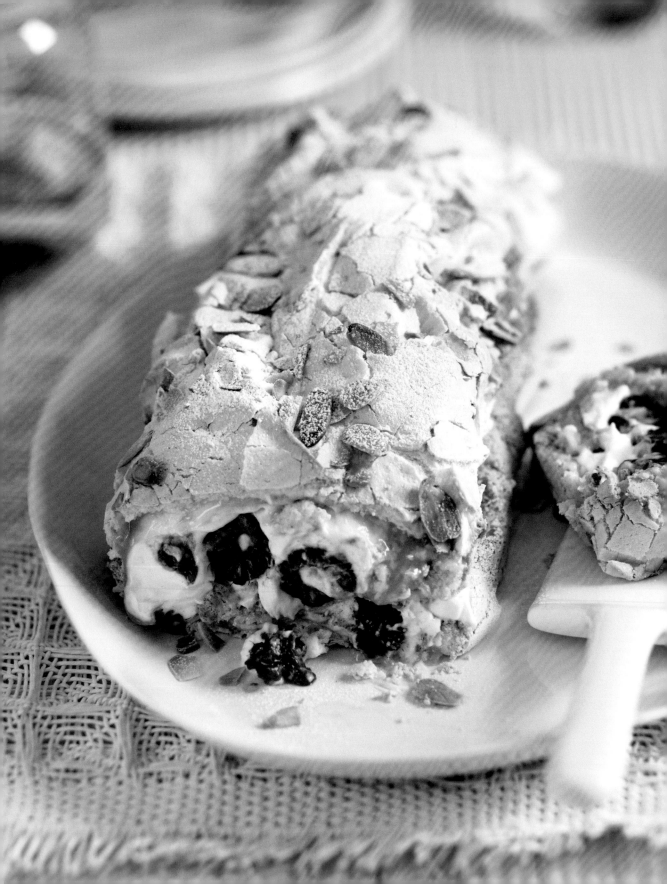

Raspberry and Lemon Curd Roulade

Serves 6-8

Ingredients

4 large organic free range eggs, separated
1¼ cups superfine sugar
2 tablespoons sliced almonds
¾ cup + 1 tablespoon heavy cream
1 x 9oz jar lemon curd
1 pint raspberries
confectioners' sugar, for dusting

Method

1. Preheat the oven to 350°F.

2. Whisk the egg whites until they start to whiten. Slowly add the sugar, 1 tablespoon at a time until they egg whites are stiff.

3. On a baking sheet lined with parchment paper, spread the egg whites with a spatula to create a ripple effect. Sprinkle with the almonds and bake for 20 minutes.

4. While the meringue is cooling, whip the cream until it holds in soft peaks and stir in the lemon curd.

5. Flip the cooled meringue onto a sheet of baking paper dusted with confectioners' sugar. Spread the cream over it and scatter with the raspberries. Roll up the roulade and serve!

*top tip
Feel free to swap the raspberries for any berry – strawberries, blueberries, and blackberries also taste great in this roulade

Roast Peaches with Passionfruit Cream and Toasted Hazelnuts

Serves 6-8

Ingredients

4 peaches, cut in half
¾ cup + 1 tablespoon heavy cream
4 passionfruit
4 tablespoons hazelnuts, toasted and crushed

Method

1. Preheat the oven to 350°F.

2. Place the peaches in an ovenproof dish and roast for approximately 20 minutes, until they begin to soften but still retain their shape. Remove from the oven and let cool slightly.

3. Whip the cream until slightly thickened. Cut the passionfruit in half and scoop out the pulp and seeds. Stir the passionfruit into the cream.

4. Arrange the peaches onto a plate, spoon the cream over the top, and scatter with the hazelnuts.

Chocolate Cheesecake Brownies

Serves 8–10

Ingredients
¾ cup + 1 tablespoon unsalted butter, melted
⅓ cup cocoa powder, sifted
½ cup superfine sugar
3 organic eggs
1¼ cups all-purpose flour, sifted
1¼ cups cream cheese, softened and chopped
4½ tablespoons superfine sugar
⅔ cup frozen raspberries

Method
1. Preheat the oven to 325°F. Line an 8in square pan with non-stick parchment paper.

2. Place the butter, cocoa, ½ cup sugar, 2 eggs, and flour in a bowl and mix well until smooth.

3. Spoon into the prepared pan.

4. Mix the cream cheese, 4½ tablespoons sugar, and remaining egg in a food processor until smooth.

5. Place the frozen raspberries on top of the chocolate mixture, then pour large spoonfuls of the cheesecake on top of the chocolate mixture and swirl with a butter knife. Bake for 45–50 minutes or until set. Let cool in the pan before cutting into squares.

*serving suggestion
Serve the crumble with some chilled full-fat plain yogurt—delicious!

Fruit Crumble

Serves 6–8

Ingredients
For the crumble
2 cups oats
1 cup walnuts
¼ cup Brazil nuts
⅓ cup almonds
½ teaspoon ground fennel seeds
¼ cup shredded coconut
2 tablespoons coconut oil
½ teaspoon cinnamon
2 tablespoons agave syrup

For the fruit
5 large organic apples, plus any other fruit you wish to add in small quantity, e.g. 2 pears
1 tablespoon coconut oil
2 tablespoons water
1 teaspoon pure vanilla extract
½ teaspoon cinnamon
2 teaspoons Manuka honey

Method
1. Preheat the oven to 350°F.

2. Make the crumble by blending all the ingredients together.

3. To make the filling, chop the fruit into small chunks. Heat the oil, water, and fruit in a pan until the fruit becomes soft, then add the vanilla, cinnamon, and honey and heat until the mixture has thickened a little.

4. Transfer to an ovenproof dish, cover with the crumble mixture, and bake in the preheated oven for around 30 minutes.

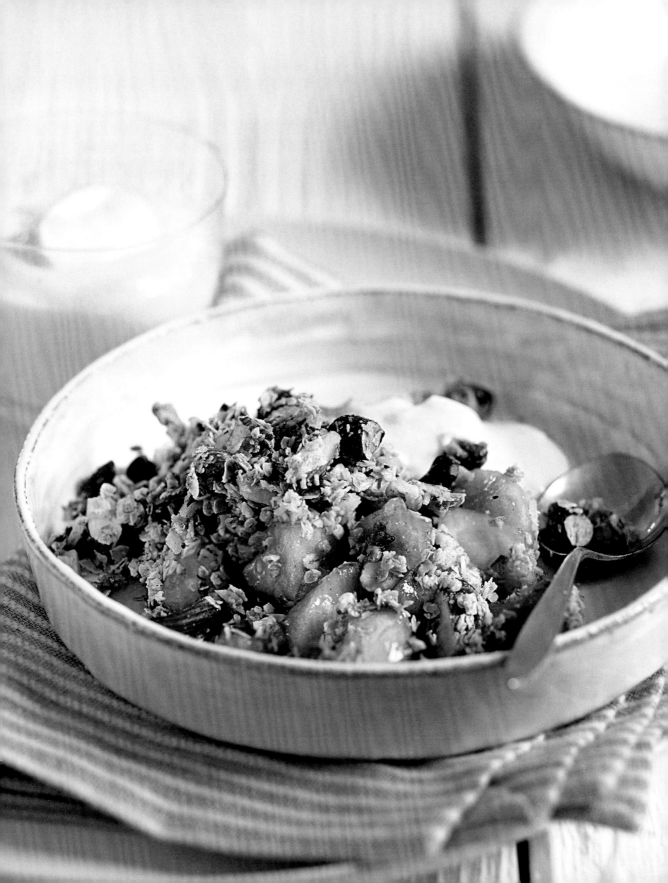

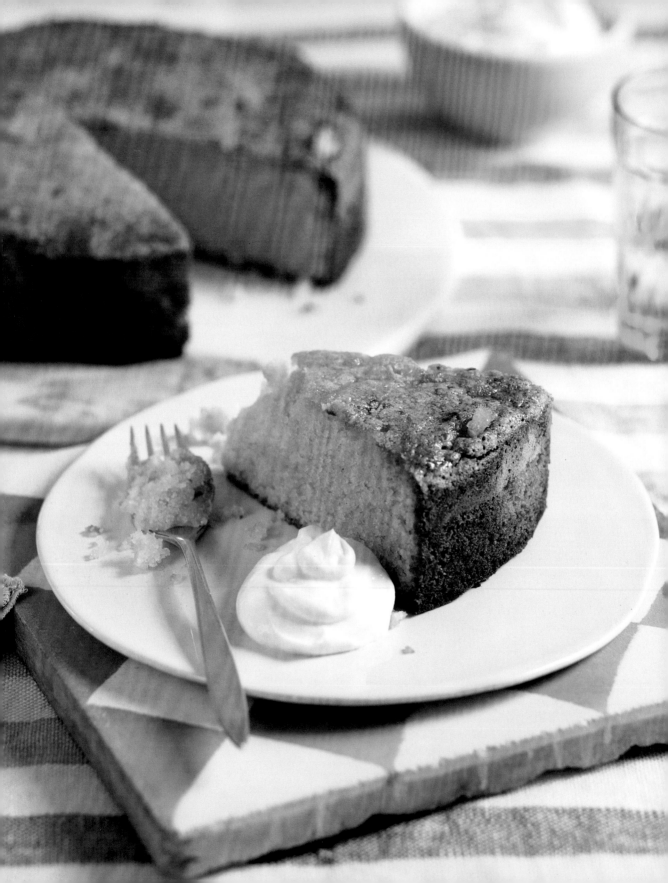

The Cupcake Company's Citrus Polenta Cake (Gluten-Free)

Serves 8

Ingredients

1½ cups almond flour
⅔ cup polenta
1 teaspoon gluten-free baking powder
4 large organic eggs, separated
¾ cup grapeseed oil
¾ cup + 1½ tablespoons superfine sugar
grated zest of 1 orange
grated zest of 1 lemon

For the syrup

⅔ cup orange juice
¼ cup superfine sugar

For the mascarpone cream topping

1 cup mascarpone
½ cup confectioners' sugar, sifted
1 cup heavy cream, whipped to soft peaks

Method

1. Preheat the oven to 350°F and lightly grease an 8in cake pan. Mix together the almond flour, polenta, and baking powder.

2. In a separate bowl, beat the egg yolks, grapeseed oil, ¾ cup superfine sugar, and orange and lemon zests until smooth. Add the dry ingredients to the egg mixture, folding gently.

3. Whisk the egg whites and the 1½ tablespoons superfine sugar in a clean bowl until stiff peaks form and add these to the cake mixture in three additions.

4. Pour into the prepared pan and bake in the center of the preheated oven for 30-35 minutes or until a skewer inserted in the center of the cake comes out clean. Let the cake cool in the pan while you make the syrup.

5. Place the orange juice and superfine sugar in a small saucepan over low heat. Stir to dissolve the sugar, bring to a boil, and boil for 1 minute. Let cool for 10 minutes.

6. Pierce the cake all over through to the bottom with a skewer, then drizzle the warm syrup over the cake. Leave for 10 minutes before turning out of the pan and let cool completely.

7. Meanwhile, make the mascarpone cream topping. Combine the mascarpone and sifted confectioners' sugar in a small bowl, then fold in the whipped cream.

8. Serve the cake with the mascarpone cream (or you can use the cream to frost the cake).

*top tip

For some extra zing, squeeze a little fresh lemon over this just before you eat it or scatter a little lemon zest over the cake or the cream to add interesting texture

HERE'S MY HANDY "BAD, BETTER & BEST"

BAD	BETTER	BEST
Bad: Chocolate cake made from a packaged mix **Why?** Packed full of sugar with no redeeming health benefits	**Better:** Homemade chocolate cake **Why?** At least you know exactly what is in it, and you can use organic ingredients if you prefer	**Best:** Homemade fruit cake with organic fruit **Why?** Contains both antioxidants and fiber
Bad: Black Forest sponge cake with ice cream **Why?** Full of flour and sugar	**Better:** Homemade Black Forest sponge cake with raspberries and cream **Why?** Raspberries are low GI	**Best:** A bowl of organic raspberries and blueberries with organic Greek yogurt **Why?** The berries are low GI and the yogurt is a good source of calcium
Bad: Fast food milkshake **Why?** A pure sugar bomb	**Better:** Homemade milkshake with fruit **Why?** The fruit contains fiber	**Best:** Organic fruit smoothie made with organic full-fat yogurt and nuts **Why?** Full of fiber and healthy fats as well as antioxidants
Bad: Ice cream sundae **Why?** Contains almost no nutrients	**Better:** Banana split with organic cream **Why?** Bananas are a good source of potassium and dietary fiber	**Best:** Slices of banana with pecans and yogurt **Why?** A balance of protein, fats, and carbohydrates
Bad: Store-bought frozen apple pie **Why?** Full of sugar and flour	**Better:** Homemade apple pie with ice cream **Why?** You know exactly what is going into it and you have the option of using organic ingredients	**Best:** Homemade organic apple pie with organic cream **Why?** Cream contains less sugar than ice cream and the pectin in apples helps lower blood cholesterol
Bad: Peanut butter shortbread **Why?** Almost no nutrient content whatsoever	**Better:** Organic peanut butter chocolate cups **Why?** Organic and contains some antioxidants	**Best:** Organic nut butter with 70 percent cocoa chocolate **Why?** Full of healthy fats and antioxidants
Bad: Eton Mess **Why?** Full of sugar with little nutritional value	**Better:** Strawberries with cream **Why?** The fruit contains nutrients but non-organic strawberries can be heavily sprayed with pesticides	**Best:** Organic cream with raspberries and sliced almonds **Why?** Quick and easy to make and full of fiber and antioxidants

DESSERTS GUIDE:

BAD	BETTER	BEST
Bad: Ice cream **Why?** Contains huge amounts of sugar. Also, many people have problems digesting dairy and this can lower the immune system and the body's ability to burn fat	**Better:** Plain organic yogurt with almonds **Why?** Contains far less sugar than ice cream and protein from the nuts helps you feel fuller for longer	**Best:** An apple and a handful of berries **Why?** Fruit is rich in antioxidants and helps detox your system
Bad: Cupcakes **Why?** Loaded with sugar, wheat, yeast, and bad fats	**Better:** Muffins from a health food shop **Why?** Contains fiber and fewer bad fats but is probably still full of fat and sugar	**Best:** Homemade muffins **Why?** You're able to see exactly what goes in them and can use gluten-free flour (cornstarch, rice flour, buckwheat, or millet) and rolled oats and antioxidant-rich berries
Bad: White sugar **Why?** Sugar is an empty food that contains almost zero health benefits, plus it's addictive	**Better:** Brown sugar **Why?** Marginally higher nutritional value than white sugar, though hardly any	**Best:** Manuka honey **Why?** Full of antioxidants, plus it also natural antibacterial, antimicrobial, antiseptic, antiviral, antioxidant, anti-inflammatory, and antifungal properties
Bad: Dried apricots **Why?** High in sugar and sulphates that destroy vitamins in the foods they preserve	**Better:** Fresh apricots **Why?** Iron-rich and a good source of fiber	**Best:** Organic apricots **Why?** No risk of sulfite exposure or any other toxin
Bad: Waxed apples **Why?** The fruit may look shiny and enticing but the wax coating drags the nutrients from the fruit	**Better:** Loose apples in a bag **Why?** More nutrient-rich. Don't peel your apples as the skin contains most of the fiber	**Best:** Organic apples **Why?** Free of any nasty toxin, even if they don't look so pretty
Bad: Instant coffee **Why?** Highly processed and full of toxins that clog up your liver. Robs your body of nutrients	**Better:** Peppermint tea **Why?** Caffeine-free and an excellent digestive aid. Try and use fresh mint leaves if possible	**Best:** Hot water with a few slices of lemon and ginger **Why?** A great detox drink and a good tip for banishing cellulite

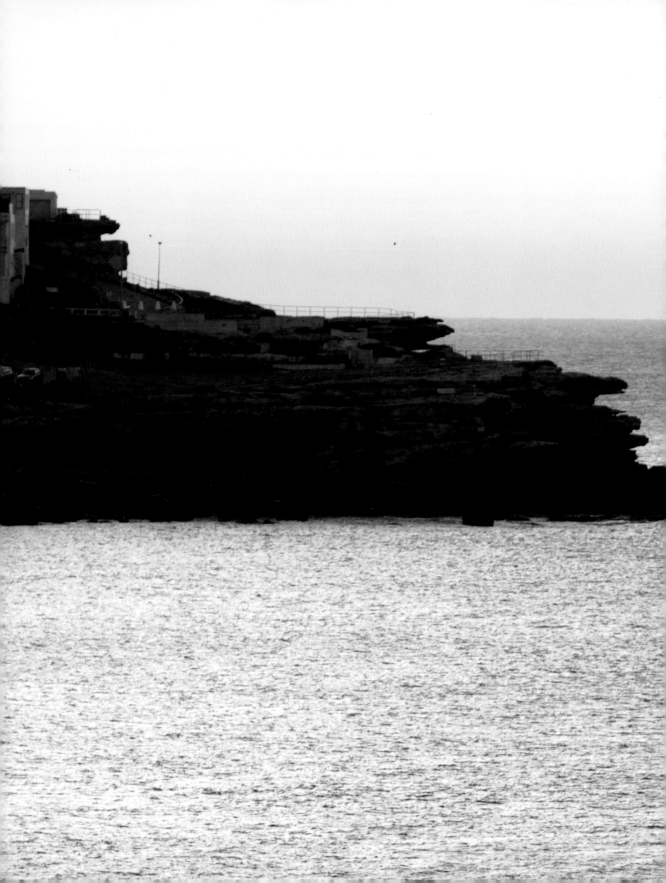

CHAPTER 8

CLEAN AND LEAN SMOOTHIES

THIS CHAPTER WILL REVEAL:

1. WHY IT'S BETTER TO BLEND

2. THE BEST FRUIT AND VEGETABLES TO USE

3. MY FAVORITE SMOOTHIE RECIPES

I'm a HUGE fan of smoothies. Both Christiane and I love them, and have them every morning. They're a fantastic way of getting a huge hit of nutrients into your body quickly and easily. When most people think of smoothies, though, they think of all-fruit concoctions. But my smoothies aren't like this. I include all kinds of foods in mine, from green vegetables to nuts and milk.

Every morning Christiane makes me an amazing green smoothie, containing anything green we happen to have in our kitchen—kale, spinach, apples, limes, cucumber, or celery. It's a great way to start the day and I know that whatever else happens throughout the rest of the day, I've had an amazing amounts of nutrients at the very start.

Why making your own is always healthier

There are a few things to keep in mind though when it comes to smoothies. Store-bought smoothies are mainly made of fruit, which makes them very high in sugar. Even the ones that contain vegetables usually contain more fruit—turn the bottles around and read the ingredients. I guarantee the top few ingredients are fruit. Store-bought smoothies are also pasteurized. This involves them going through a heating process—it keeps them safe as it keeps them from spoiling quickly—but it also destroys a lot of the health-boosting nutrients found in the fruits and vegetables. So where possible, always make your own.

It's better to blend

In the last few years there has also been a move away from "juicing" to "blending." When you juice ingredients, you mix them until they're a very smooth consistency. When you blend them, you leave them a little chunkier. The latter option is much healthier because digestion starts with chewing. When you drink a very smooth smoothie, your body doesn't really work to digest it and over time this can make your digestive system lazy. But when you chew chunks from your smoothie, your digestive system fires up and works harder to process what you're swallowing. The pulp and fiber in a chunkier smoothie is better for your system. So in a nutshell, try to make your "smoothies" a little less smooth and a little more chunky.

Lastly, don't treat a smoothie as a "drink." It isn't—it's either a meal (say, in the case of breakfast, if it contains nuts and other ingredients that make it calorific enough for breakfast) or a snack. If you treat it as a drink—especially a mainly fruit-based smoothie—you'll take in a lot of calories on top of your meals without realizing.

Supercharge your smoothie:

✳ Add a handful of nuts to up the protein content of your smoothie. Protein keeps your metabolism fired up and it keeps you full for hours.
✳ Add lots of ice—avoid topping off with sugary juices and throw in some ice-cubes instead.
✳ Add some supplements. I always add BodyBrilliance to mine (go to www.bodyism.com).
✳ Add some chopped herbs, like mint. They'll improve the flavor and add health benefits too.
*Lastly, always drink your smoothie with a straw—prolonged contact with fruit sugars can damage your teeth.

The best fruit and vegetables to blend in a smoothie

FRUIT	VEGETABLES
✳ Blueberries	✳ Celery
✳ Apples	✳ Kale
✳ Pomegranates	✳ Spinach
✳ Oranges	✳ Green beans
✳ Plums	✳ Asparagus
✳ Kiwis	✳ Zucchini
✳ Mangoes	✳ Broccoli
✳ Bananas	✳ Peas
✳ Pineapples	✳ Bok choy
✳ Cranberries	✳ Beets
✳ Lemons	✳ Bell peppers
✳ Blackberries	
✳ Strawberries	
✳ Raspberries	

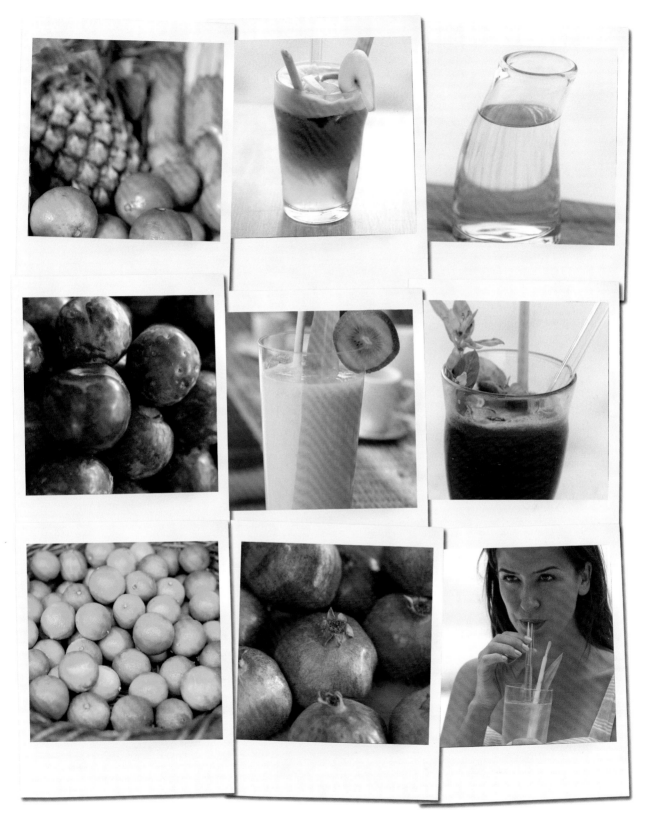

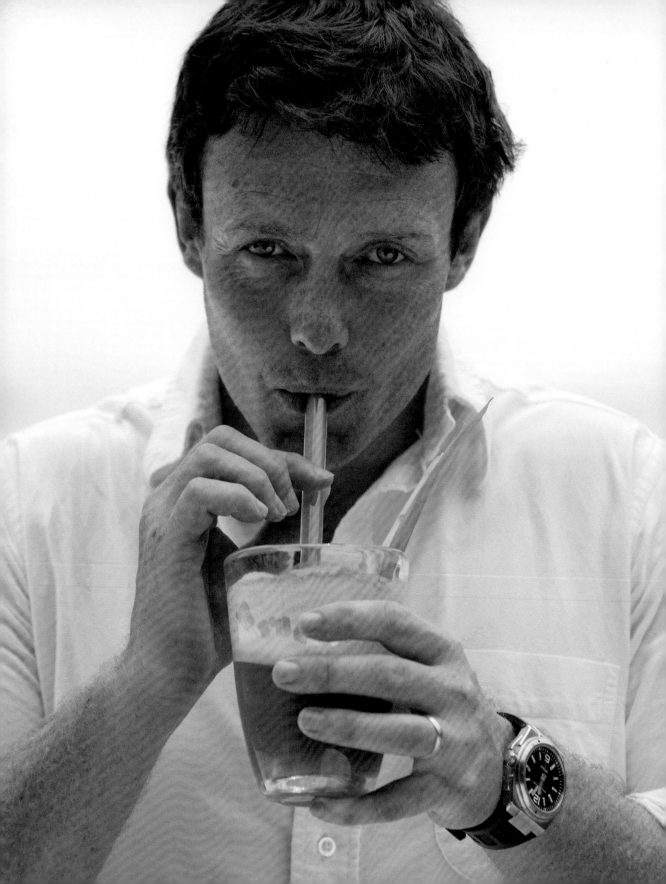

Detox Smoothie

Serves 1

Ingredients

1 scoop Bodyism Greens
1 cup coconut water
1 teaspoon mint
1 celery rib
1 teaspoon grated ginger
2 large handfuls of spinach
½ cucumber
½ apple

Method

Blend all the ingredients together and serve immediately.

The Nourisher

Serves 1

Ingredients

½ teaspoon cinnamon
¼ cup blueberries
¾ cup Greek yogurt
1 tablespoon unsweetened coconut flakes or 1 teaspoon coconut oil
ice

Method

Blend all the ingredients together and serve immediately.

Breakfast Smoothie

Serves 1

Ingredients

1 scoop Bodyism BodyBrilliance
1 scoop Bodyism UltimateClean Fibre
2 Brazil nuts
¼ cup blueberries
1 tablespoon ground flax
¾ cup rice milk

Method

Blend all the ingredients together and serve immediately.

*top tip

All Bodyism supplements are available at www.bodyism.com

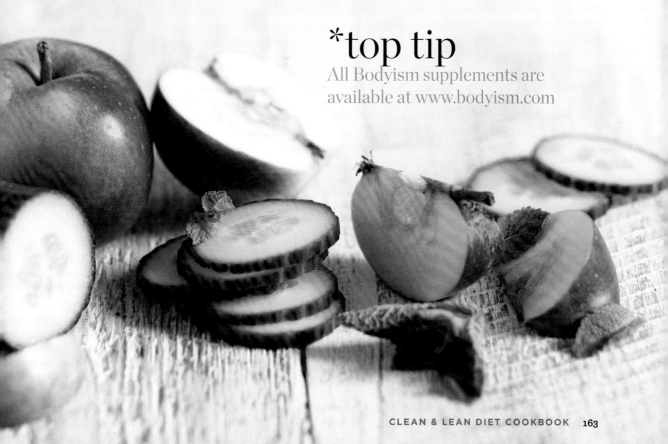

Berry Smoothie

Serves 1

Ingredients
1 tablespoon blueberries
1 tablespoon strawberries
1 tablespoon blackberries
1 tablespoon raspberries
½ cup natural yogurt
½ teaspoon cinnamon
½ cup rice milk

Method
Blend all the ingredients together
and serve immediately.

Indulgent Shake

Serves 1

Ingredients
1 scoop Bodyism BodyComplete
2 drops vanilla extract
½ teaspoon cinnamon
2 Brazil nuts
2 tablespoons peanut butter

Method
Blend all the ingredients together
and serve immediately.

S&M Greens

Serves 1

Ingredients
a handful of spinach
a handful of broccoli
¼ cucumber
1 teaspoon grated ginger
1 celery rib
squeeze of lemon
½ cup water

Method
Blend all the ingredients
together and serve
immediately.

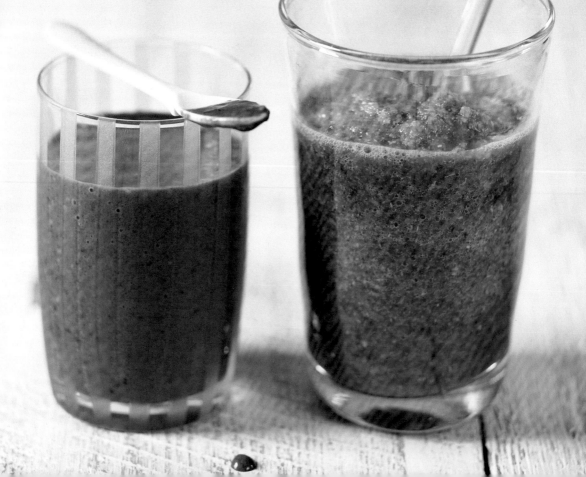

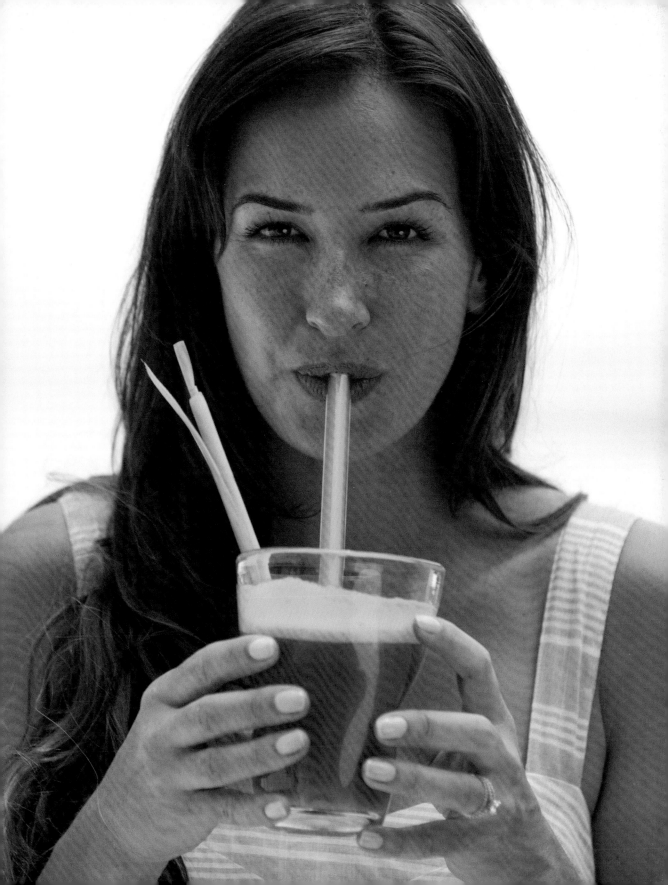

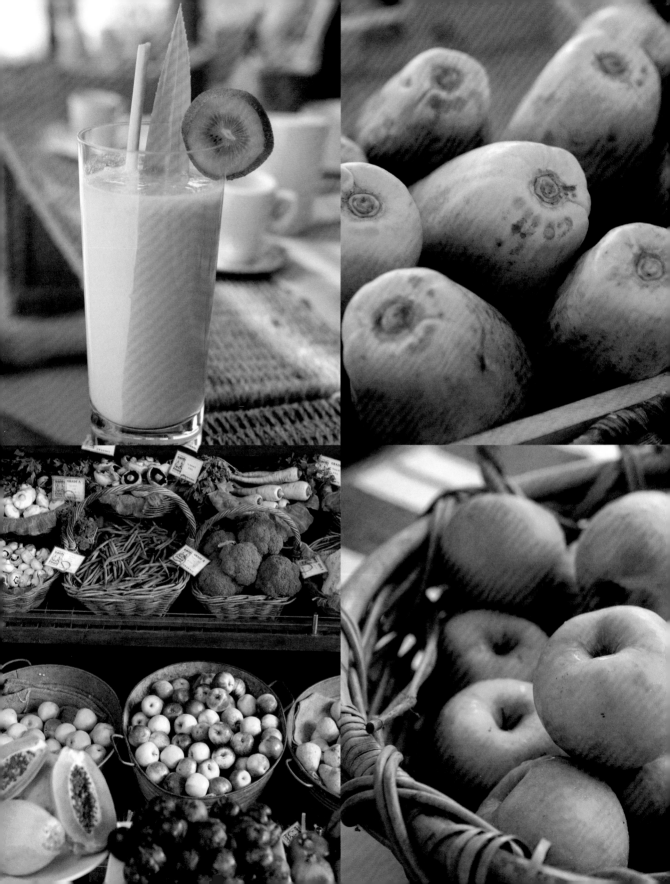

Ultimate Complete Shake

Serves 1

Ingredients
1 scoop Bodyism BodyBrilliance
1 scoop Bodyism BodyComplete
1 scoop Bodyism UltimateClean Fibre
1 scoop Bodyism Greens

Method
Blend all the ingredients together and serve immediately.

Izzy's Shake

Serves 4

Ingredients
1 banana
½ ripe avocado
1 tablespoon green spirulina powder
1 tablespoon chlorella
1 tablespoon maca powder
2 tablespoons ground flaxseed
goji berries, optional
1 tablespoon coconut flour, optional
1 tablespoon activated chia seeds, soaked in water overnight
1 tablespoon bee pollen
6 Brazil nuts
11 teaspoons cinnamon
2–3 tablespoons protein powder
1 tablespoon unsweetened cocoa
1 tablespoon honey
1 cup unsweetened almond milk
3 cups filtered water
1 tablespoon Acai syrup

Method
Blend all the ingredients together and serve immediately.

Morning Booster Shake

Serves 1

Ingredients
8fl oz water or milk
1 scoop BodyBrilliance
1 scoop UltimateClean Fibre
3 Brazil nuts
a handful of sunflower seeds
a handful of pumpkin seeds
a pinch of turmeric

Method
Blend all the ingredients together and serve immediately.

Lean Physic Shake

Serves 1

Ingredients
1 scoop Bodyism BodyComplete
1 cup rice milk or almond milk
1 scoop lecithin
½ scoop Bodyism BeautyFood, optional

Method
Blend all the ingredients together and serve immediately.

*top tip
You don't have to stick to these ingredients—try adding your favorite clean and lean ingredients to your smoothies

Bodyism
Bloody Mary

Serves 1

Ingredients
⅔ cup tomato juice
1 celery rib
¼ cucumber
a pinch of black pepper
ice

Method
Blend all the ingredients together
and serve immediately.

Good Night's
Sleep

Serves 1

Ingredients
1 scoop Bodyism Serenity
¾ cup vanilla rice milk
8 cashews

Method
Blend all the ingredients together
and serve immediately.

Anti-aging
Smoothie

Serves 1

Ingredients
3fl oz water
½ cucumber
½ avocado
1 celery rib
squeeze of lemon juice
a small handful of green leaves or
1 scoop Bodyism BeautyFood
1 teaspoon grated ginger

Method
Blend all the ingredients together
and serve immediately.

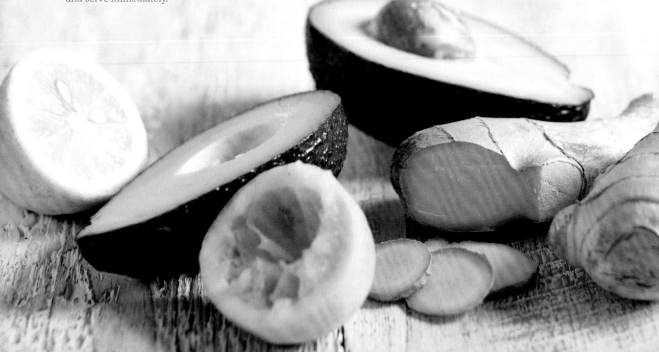

Super Green Smoothie

Serves 1

Ingredients
1 cup water
1 scoop Bodyism BeautyFood
juice of 1 lemon or lime
5 mint leaves
2 slices of ginger

Method
Blend all the ingredients together
and serve immediately.

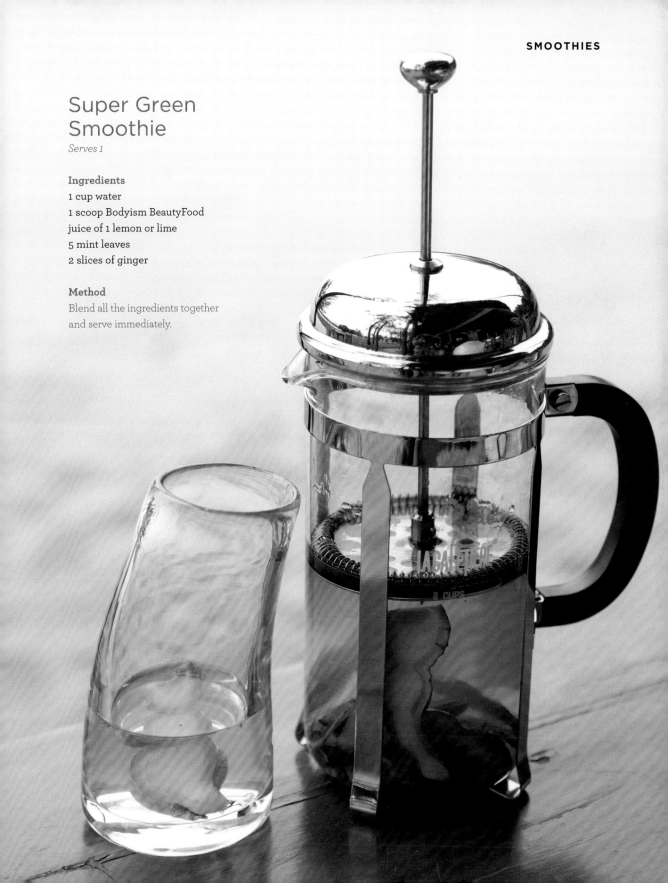

INDEX

MY CLIENTS

People often ask me what Elle Macpherson is really like, so I thought I'd tell you a few things about her you may not know. From the first time I met her, she has never stopped helping me. In fact, she's always looking for ways in which she can be of service to the people in her life. She's the hardest worker I know, and yet she always makes time for the people she loves. She's also very generous—in all the years I have known her she has never once asked for anything in return, ever. She always asks about my family, which is such a lovely and easy thing to do, but not something everyone does, and whenever she has anything she always looks to share it. She loves her children and she's proud of them, too, and when she talks about them she lights up. She always looks for the positive in a situation and in a person. She never gossips, complains, gives up, or looks for excuses, which are all such amazing qualities. She's highly principled too. Whenever I have a new project I want her advice on, her first questions are always about its integrity. It's never about how much money she could make but whether she believes in what is being done. But perhaps the most profound impact Elle has had on my life is this: when I first met my wife, Christiane, I loved her from the moment I saw her, but it took me a while to get the courage to ask her to marry me. It was a Monday when Elle walked into the gym, She asked me how things were and how was Christiane. "Fine," I said. "So when are you going to ask her to marry you?" I replied I was nervous and scared, etc., etc. Elle put her hands on my shoulders, looked me straight in the eye and said the following: "Christiane is a beautiful person, inside and out. She will be an amazing mother and a best friend to you forever. You love her and she loves you. Ask this woman to marry you and let go of being scared." So I did, and she said yes! And I'm so thankful every single day that I have such an amazing wife and a friend who cared enough to tell it to me straight. I'll stop there, but I hope you get the picture. She's one amazing lady.

People also ask me what Rosie Huntington-Whiteley is like in "real life" and I can only say this. She is also one of the most remarkable, highly principled, and generous people I have ever met and I'm still astonished at what an amazing and humble person she is. She's beautiful on the inside and obviously on the outside. I once asked her why she is so supportive of me and her answer was typically inspiring, brilliant, and honest. She said, "Because I believe in what you're saying and what you're trying to do. I really do support you and I want to help do something good." I just think it's great that she has the courage of her convictions and that she constantly thinks of how she can help others. Rosie is one in a million. She's someone that I love and admire, that I can count on as a friend no matter what, which is pretty cool in my opinion. Just be careful if you ever have breakfast with her—she will eat all your granola!

People also ask me about Hugh Grant. He has become a really good friend of mine over the years and I love him very much. I just want to share a little story about him that might give you insight into the kind and beautiful person he is. A few years ago, one of our trainers became ill. I paid the medical bills, but it started to get really expensive and was becoming more than I could afford. Hugh knew about the situation but hadn't really said much about it other than to ask how things were going. As the months went by we all got increasingly concerned and worried. Hugh was just about to go off for a while filming but he came in to Bodyism the day he left to say goodbye. As he left, he handed me a blank check and said, "Make sure she gets whatever she needs. It doesn't matter what it costs." That's the kind of man Hugh Grant is. That's what he is like in real life and I love him for it. As he walked out he also said, "Please don't spend it on a sex change." Which is also why I love him. He might be angry at me for telling this story but I don't care. I want people to know what a kind-hearted person he really is. (Our lovely trainer is completely healthy now by the way!)

Finally, I just want to quickly mention my amazing, wonderful, and beautiful friend David de Rothschild. He has inspired me to do more and to be more. He gave me a bigger problem to tackle, to help as many people in the world as I can. Please log on to myoo.com to see how you can help too.

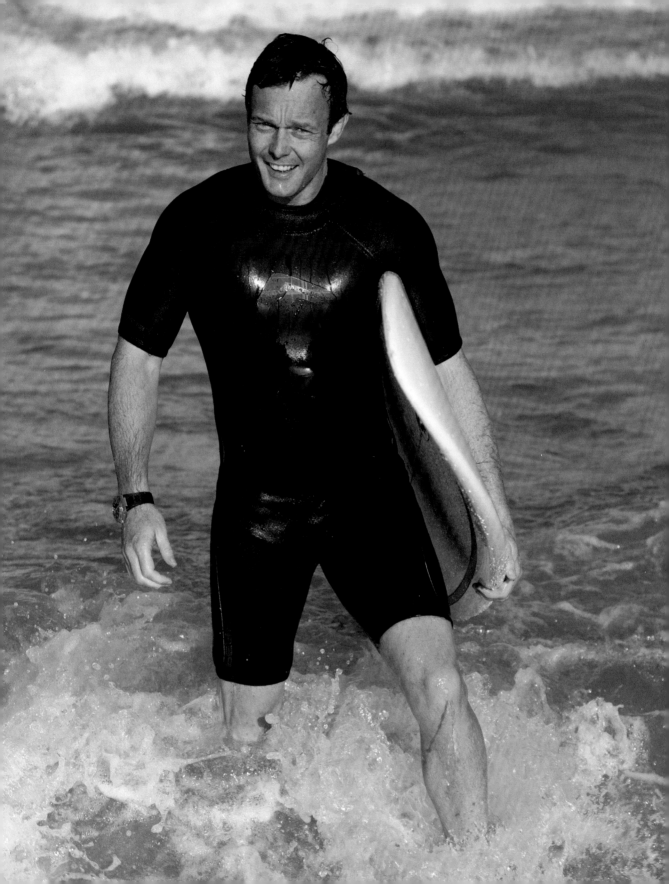

ACKNOWLEDGEMENTS

I'd like to **thank** the following people for making this book possible. Firstly my wife, Christiane. I love you more and more every day, you were the **driving** force of this book, and your **ideas** and passion are what make these things **special** and amazing. I love that you're smarter than me and I love having you on my team. You're my **best** friend and I love every bit of you in every way. Thank you for your **beautiful** heart. Elle, Rosie, and Hugh, thank you for **everything**. To Zoe Kravitz, you're like a little sister to me and I love you very much, you're such a wonderful person and me and my amore miss you lots. You're kind, **generous,** and special and I can't wait to see the amazing things you do in this world. Unleash your inner warrior **goddess**! To Holly Valance, I'm a better dancer than you but you're quite funny. You're also a **warm**, generous, and caring **soul** and Christiane and I both think you're the best and we love spending time with you, thank you again for being so cool. To Lee for staying **awake** and helping me on that long last night before deadline. You invented some very interesting foods and your **support** is something I will never forget, I **love** you. To David de Rothschild, for inspiring me and **believing** in me and for being a big beautiful friend that gives me hugs, I love you. To Sebastian and Emily for taking such beautiful photos and being such wonderful friends. To Linda for being so incredibly **incredible**, I can't put into words how **grateful** I am to you and how much I admire you. To Nat for being so amazing, brilliant, and such a huge part of all that we do. To Clara, Megan, Michelle, (and Toby and Cupcake and Bud Bud) for the **wonderful** recipes and beautiful friendship. To Dalton, for driving us home from bjj when I'm dizzy and for having the **courage** to evolve, it's amazing. To my friend Justin Alexander, OG. To my mom and dad, the best people I know and to my little sister, I'm so **proud** of you. And to Chantal and Luke and Sol, for making it all **possible** and for being such beautiful friends. We love you all so much! To my wonderful publishers, thank you Kyle and Judith and Vicki! Tommy, I literally don't know what I would do without you, **definitely** not horse riding. **Thank you** Maria.... we did it again, even better!

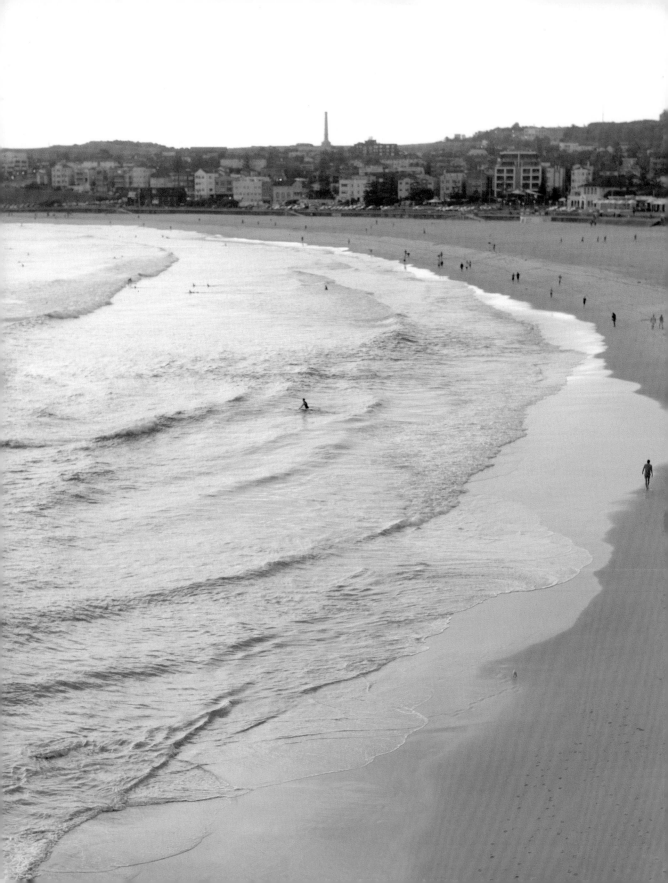